MENOPAUSE MAKEOVER: TRANSFORMING YOUR LIFE

LISA M. CARROLL

NYC Girl LLC

CONTENTS

First Edition 2023

INTRODUCTION

Life has a funny way of presenting the most significant transformations to us, doesn't it? Right when you've waved your child off to college when you've finally nailed that crow pose in yoga, or found your favorite wine after countless trials and errors, a knock resounds on the door. "Who's there?" you might ask. "It's me, Menopause," replies a voice full of unwavering certainty. Menopause is an uninvited yet inevitable visitor, making itself comfortable in your life, much like an old friend bearing gifts wrapped in mystery and challenge.

My name is Lisa, and I'm all too familiar with the nuances of this 'old friend.' As a professional navigating the complex labyrinth of life in my fifties, I've made it my mission to understand this transition that nature has in store for every woman. Over the last decade, my journey through perimenopause and menopause has been filled with laughter, frustration, contemplation, a bigger waistline, and, most importantly, revelation. And here I am, extending my hand to you as an ally, as a fellow traveler who's walked a few steps ahead, clearing the path for a smoother journey for you.

Menopause is a crossroads, a time of profound metamorphosis. It's a time when the body whispers, sometimes screams, echoing the changes happening within. I know the frustration of feeling like a stranger in your own body. I also know the courage it takes to seek answers, to learn, to adapt, and to reclaim one's power. This book is born from my experience, my struggles, my victories, and my incessant quest for knowledge and answers. It is an embodiment of my desire to ensure that no woman ever feels alone or misunderstood during this phase.

Picture this book as a warm, nurturing conversation between friends, mingling the practical with the profound, the scientific with the experiential. Through these pages, I aim to arm you with the knowledge and strategies to thrive during menopause, quell anxieties, and embrace the change with grace and grit. I'll share the lessons I've learned, the tips that have worked, the myths I've debunked, and the discoveries that have made me say, "Aha!"

So, why should you trust this book? Because I've lived the confusion, weathered the hot flashes, and asked the questions that kept me awake at 3 am. I've experimented, I've learned, and I've gathered all those pearls of wisdom right here for you.

This book will guide you through understanding the whirlwind that is menopause, decode its effects on your body and mind, and equip you with practical, effective strategies to manage the symptoms. It's a treasure trove of insights to help you redefine menopause from a daunting change into a journey of empowerment and self-discovery.

The journey of menopause is not simply about survival but about flourishing. It's a chapter of your life waiting to be written with bravery, laughter, wisdom, and, yes, the occasional hot flash. Are you ready to redefine your menopause story? Let's dive in, one page at a time!

PROLOGUE

Welcome to a series of real stories, tales of lives lived, and experiences earned, all collected from the women who inspired me to write this book. The narratives you are about to read are not fabricated or drawn from an imaginative realm. They are true, they are raw, and they are the realities of women from all walks of life.

Each story you will find in this book emerged from personal conversations, interviews, and heart-to-heart discussions. They delve into the subject of women's health, but not just from a clinical or scientific perspective. These stories expose the human side of the coin, the side that often gets left out when discussing health and science.

To protect their privacy, I have changed the names and certain identifying details of these brave women. However, I have tried to preserve the essence of their experiences, keeping their stories as authentic as when they were first shared with me.

Beyond the scientific knowledge we will explore, these narratives will offer a learning experience from a unique standpoint:

human resilience, strength, and perseverance. They remind us that there's more to health than just science; there's also the human experience.

I am deeply grateful to these women for sharing their journeys with me and allowing me to share them with you. As you turn the pages, I invite you to learn from their experiences, appreciate their courage, and explore the human side of science. These stories are not just narratives; they are real-life lessons and inspirations.

The Silent Nightmare

Sarah was just an ordinary woman living an ordinary life. Until one day, she wasn't. Without warning, she found herself grappling with intense migraines, an inexplicable weight gain, and hot flashes as fierce as midsummer heat waves. Menopause, a silent intruder, had invaded her life.

Sarah was puzzled and scared. The aches and hot flashes were hard enough, but the uncertainty was the worst part. She spent countless hours Googling her symptoms, each search promising a grim diagnosis. From rare brain disorders to incurable diseases, the internet seemed determined to convince her that the end was near.

With each passing day, her anxiety grew. It felt like a secret ticking time bomb was nestled within her. She was too young for this, she thought. It didn't make sense. It felt like she was on an unending roller-coaster, with no sight of when it would stop.

To distract herself from this whirlwind of worry, Sarah decided to join a local yoga class. Yoga, she hoped, might calm her body and mind. At the very least, it was a welcome distraction from the dizzying array of possible ailments she found online.

One afternoon, mid-way through a Downward Dog pose, the yoga instructor said, "This pose is great for menopause symptoms - hot flashes, migraines, even mood swings."

Menopause? The word hit her like a revelation. She had been so wrapped up in fears of rare diseases she had completely overlooked something so common yet life-altering. As the instructor moved on to the next pose, Sarah stayed still, suspended in the sudden clarity, with a cartoon "a-ha" above her head.

"The Silent Nightmare" was not silent anymore. It was just menopause, something millions of women experience. It wasn't a death sentence; it was just a natural part of life. And with that realization, Sarah couldn't help but burst out laughing right there in the middle of the yoga studio. Her laughter echoed through the quiet room, a testament to her relief, a symbol of her newfound understanding and acceptance of the journey ahead.

Red Rage and Revelation

In a bustling city filled with towering skyscrapers and countless dreams, there lived a woman whose life was upended by a crimson storm. Unnamed and unacknowledged, it swept through her life, leaving in its wake chaos that she had never known before. Let's call her Rachel.

Rachel was no stranger to life's ups and downs, but this, this was something different. A creeping malaise that colored her days with inexplicable fits of fury, punctuated by emotional whirlwinds that spun her life out of control. Little did she know, she was in the throes of an invisible tempest – the onset of perimenopause.

In a world that prizes youth and dismisses the signs of its fading, Rachel's pleas were met with disregard and disdain.

"You're too young," the doctors would say, patting her arm reassuringly while they tossed her concerns aside. They saw a woman who was too young to be grappling with such issues, while Rachel saw a reflection in the mirror that seemed increasingly alien to her.

Ensnared in a vicious cycle of unexplained anger and emotional tumult, she felt like a ship lost in a stormy sea with no lighthouse to guide her. But Rachel was made of stronger stuff. She decided to take the reins of her life back into her hands.

One day, in the throngs of yet another dismissal, she chose to turn away from the familiar path and chart her own course. She started her hunt for a doctor who would listen, who would acknowledge her struggle, and validate her fight.

Her journey was not without its hardships. It was like searching for a needle in a haystack. But every 'no' brought her closer to the 'yes' she was seeking. Until one day, she found it - a medical professional who finally looked past her age and into her soul. She was diagnosed with perimenopause, a revelation that brought about a sense of vindication and relief.

Rachel's life took a sharp turn as she stepped onto the path of hormone replacement therapy. Each pill, each injection, was like a piece of a puzzle that gradually started putting her life back together. Her tempestuous moods began to calm, her uncontrollable anger subdued, replaced by a newfound sense of control and balance.

But the transformation didn't stop at her personal life. As she reclaimed control over her emotions, Rachel found the courage to break through her professional glass ceiling. She grew from strength to strength, shattering barriers and outpacing expectations.

Ageless Fire

In a world where silence and struggle were synonyms lived a heroine named Linda. Now, don't get the wrong idea. She didn't slay dragons or possess supernatural powers. Linda's adversaries were far more elusive, hidden within the labyrinth of her own body - formidable opponents named hormonal imbalances and obstinate fibroids.

Imagine, if you will, the discomfort of a hot summer's day, then amplify that a hundredfold. That was the furnace Linda contended with daily, a fierce hot flash that engulfed her without warning. Then there were the mood swings, drastic and unpredictable, tossing her between laughter and tears like a ship in a tempest. The migraines, oh, those were the traitors, silent but debilitating, attacking when least expected.

For many, this was an irrevocable curse, but not for Linda. Our heroine decided to take matters into her own hands, turning her struggles into her motivation.

One day, she descended into the catacombs of medical literature, arming herself with knowledge. Each page she turned, each piece of information she gathered, was a step closer to understanding the mysterious maze of her body. This wasn't easy. Many a night, she'd fight off sleep, her weary eyes glued to medical articles, seeking solace in the world of academia.

Linda's quest led her to a revelation - the power of lifestyle changes. It started subtly, a salad replacing a cheeseburger, water triumphing over soda, and steps chosen over escalators. Next came yoga and meditation, two allies she embraced in her battle. As she held each pose and breathed each mindful breath, she could feel the tides turning.

But it wasn't all about yoga mats and organic food. Linda enlisted the help of modern medicine, a battalion of tiny white pills. Each pill she swallowed was a bullet aimed at her tormentors, gradually bringing her body back under her command.

Throughout this journey, something magical happened. Linda began to change, not just physically but emotionally. She discovered self-acceptance, a treasure more valuable than any pill or yoga pose. She learned to view her body not as an enemy but as a part of her identity.

She began to see menopause not as a sign of aging but as a symbol of her relentless spirit, her indomitable will. It was a badge of honor she wore proudly, a testament to the ageless fire within her.

My Tryst With Menopause

You've journeyed with me through the personal narratives of incredible women, each battling their own tempest in the realm of hormones. Now, I invite you into my world, my chaos, my own personal struggle.

There I was, dressed in my United States Air Force Service Dress or Blues uniform, a lone woman surrounded by a fortress of male officers and civilian colleagues. The room was dominated by a giant conference table, around which were seated no less than fifteen individuals, including my boss, a 3-Star General. The air in the room was thick with anticipation as my turn to brief approached.

Suddenly, a strange warmth began to invade my body. It was not the kind of warmth you feel on a sunny day. It was a scorching sensation as if my blood was boiling in my veins. I looked around, expecting others to comment on the apparent heatwave, but all I encountered were indifferent faces.

The thermostat hadn't gone wild. I had.

My heart pounded like a war drum in my chest. Was it a heart attack? But there was no numbness, no tingling sensation. As beads of sweat began to race down my back, I was seized by a feeling of helplessness. I couldn't flee; my turn to brief was approaching. The heat wave eventually subsided after what felt like an eternity. That was my introduction to the world of 'hot flashes,' the first of many that would invade my life.

Following that day, my body seemed to embark on a rebellion of its own. I started having periods so heavy they could have been a scene out of a horror film, tormenting me for 10-15 days at a stretch, allowing me a breather for only a week or two before the onslaught began anew. The supposed remedy, endometrial ablation and removal of a fibroid which promised to put an end to my periods proved futile against my bodily mutiny.

My nights were no longer about rest. Hot flashes and night sweats turned my bed into an ocean, forcing me to surrender my sleep and take midnight showers. Exhaustion clung to me like a second skin, and my mind felt as if it were wading through a dense fog. I was beginning to lose myself to an unseen enemy.

I reached out to doctors, hoping for relief, only to be turned away. Their dismissive words echoed in my ears - "Everyone goes through it" - a heartless mantra repeated by five different doctors, three of them women. It felt as though I was trapped in a labyrinth of suffering with no way out.

In my desperation, I turned to the world of supplements. Magnesium became my lifeline, helping me reclaim some sleep and energy. It empowered me to return to exercise, a lifelong habit I just could not get myself to do. This helped me to regain a semblance of control over my own body. And then came testosterone pellet treatment - my ultimate game-changer.

Yet, my journey is far from over. I still face the unpredictability of sporadic periods every 10-11 months. But through it all, I've discovered important lessons. I've learned to be my own advocate, to trust in my strength, and to never accept dismissive answers. I've learned that the path to health and well-being is not a straight line but a labyrinth filled with challenges, discoveries, and moments of triumph. Alan Watts once said, "The only way to make sense out of change is to plunge into it, move with it, and join the dance."

And so, I keep dancing.

THE PERIMENOPAUSE PARADOX: EMBRACING THE UNEXPECTED

"Perimenopause." Now there's a word that could win you a game of Scrabble.

But outside the game board, it seems like a complicated mess. Is it a rare bird species? A Greek island, perhaps? No, it's neither. It's a term that sums up a cocktail of fluctuating hormones, unpredictable periods, and mood swings that would give a roller coaster a run for its money. Welcome to the world of women's health!

Alright, enough fancy terms. Let's talk about what we're about to dive into. This chapter is like a navigational guide through the labyrinth of perimenopause. It's the equivalent of having a chat with a wise, humorous, and slightly nerdy friend who happens to be a women's health aficionado.

First, we'll make sure we're all on the same page about what perimenopause really is. It's a term bandied about so much you'd think it was a new line of designer handbags. We'll unveil the mystery, breaking it down like a Lego set. We'll then dive into the thrilling world of hormones - primarily our star player, estrogen, who decides to play hardball during peri-menopause. We'll explore her fluctuating moods and how she basically decides to turn your body into her personal amusement park.

If there's one thing to be assured of, it's that this journey through perimenopause is not going to be a snore-fest. Think of it as a fascinating voyage through your body's inner workings, full of twists and turns that even Agatha Christie couldn't dream up. So, brace yourself as we unmask perimenopause, one hot flash at a time.

UNDERSTANDING PERIMENOPAUSE

So, what is this mystical term 'Perimenopause'?

The root 'peri' is a Greek prefix meaning 'around' or 'near,' while 'menopause' is that much-dreaded moment when menstruation says its final adieu. So, in simple terms, 'perimenopause' is the twilight phase around menopause; it's the red carpet event leading up to the grand premiere. It's that blurry space where you aren't quite "old," but your ovaries have started penning their retirement letters.

During this stage, the ovaries start acting a little, well, unpredictable. They're like that one friend we all have who can't decide where to eat. One day they're all about producing eggs and hormones; the next, they're like, "Nah, I'm good." This hormonal hokey pokey can lead to changes in menstrual cycle length and flow and can trigger symptoms like hot flashes, sleep disturbances, mood changes, and more.

Imagine your body is a well-tuned orchestra, with the reproductive hormones playing a harmonious symphony. When perimenopause arrives, it's as though the conductor went on break, leaving the musicians—your hormones—to play without guidance. The result is a period of discordant music that can last anywhere from a few years to a decade.

The symptoms of perimenopause are largely due to this fluctuation and gradual decrease in hormones, specifically estrogen and progesterone. They vary widely among women, so there's no 'standard' perimenopause experience. It's kind of like every woman gets a customized trip through this hormonal theme park, with rides ranging from 'mildly inconvenient' to 'oh dear god, why.'

But hey, this isn't a cause for panic or a reason to order a lifetime supply of chocolate ice cream (though no judgment if you do). Understanding what perimenopause is and what to expect during this stage can help you better manage this phase of life. In essence, perimenopause is your body's way of saying, "Heads up! Things are changing." And with the right information, you can say back, "No problem, body. I've got this!"

DIFFERENCE BETWEEN PERIMENOPAUSE AND MENOPAUSE

Let's think about it this way: if the reproductive years were a long-running TV series (with your menstrual cycle playing the lead, naturally), then perimenopause would be like those thrilling final seasons leading up to the grand finale. Meanwhile, menopause is the dramatic, confetti-filled season finale itself, wrapping up the storylines and signifying the end of the menstrual programming.

During perimenopause, the body's production of estrogen and progesterone, the key hormones in a woman's reproductive cycle, starts to fluctuate. It's like the hormones are throwing their own retirement party, and the consequences of this are irregular periods, hot flashes, mood swings, and other delightful symptoms. Think of it as your body's hormonal roller coaster ride before the park closes.

Menopause, in contrast, is the point where the period party officially ends – it is diagnosed retrospectively after a woman has missed her periods for 12 consecutive months. It's as if your body finally sends out the memo: "Folks, the reproductive factory is officially closed. No more periods. Pack up!"

While the symptoms of perimenopause and menopause can be similar, they vary in frequency and intensity. Perimenopause can sometimes feel like a hormonal tempest, with symptoms appearing suddenly and inconsistently. Menopause, on the other hand, is more like the calm after the storm. The symptoms, though still present, tend to decrease in severity over time. Imagine it like having survived a storm, and now you're just dealing with the occasional gusts of wind.

Let's talk timelines. Perimenopause can start as early as your mid-30s or as late as your 50s, though the average age is around mid-40s. It's not an overnight process; perimenopause is a marathon, not a sprint, typically lasting for several years. Menopause, however, has a more precise time frame. The average age for women to reach menopause is 51, although this can vary.

So, think of perimenopause as the pre-game show and menopause as the main event. Both are important parts of the process and are as normal as every other bodily function – just with more fanfare!

THE ROLE OF ESTROGEN

Hold onto your seats, folks, as we're about to be introduced to the reigning queen of our hormonal symphony - the melodious, magnanimous, but sometimes maddeningly mercurial -

Estrogen. If perimenopause was an opera, she'd be the lead soprano, belting out high notes one moment and leaving us in suspenseful silence the next. So get your opera glasses ready because we're diving into the intricacies of this powerhouse hormone, her mood swings, and her unforgettable solos that dictate the pace of perimenopause.

Fluctuations of estrogen during perimenopause

Next up on our tour of the hormonal hall of fame is the diva herself: estrogen. Now, if hormones were a band, estrogen would be the lead vocalist - the Beyonce of your body, if you will. She sets the rhythm for the reproductive system, overseeing everything from your periods to your mood swings.

But during perimenopause, estrogen gets temperamental. Picture her as a rockstar on a world tour, belting out chart-toppers one day and then deciding to skip the next few concerts because she didn't like the hotel's room service. Estrogen levels fluctuate wildly during perimenopause, causing a cascade of changes in the body.

It's like a hormonal game of 'Chutes and Ladders.' One moment, you're cruising smoothly, and then you hit a chute (a plunge in estrogen), and suddenly you're dealing with hot flashes, sleep disturbances, and mood changes. But then, estrogen spikes, and it feels like you've climbed a ladder, only to land on another chute as the cycle repeats. Welcome to the estrogen rollercoaster!

The link between estrogen and reproductive years

Now, let's do a little time travel. Back to when you hit puberty, and estrogen first entered the scene, turning you from a girl into a woman. From then on, she's been the puppet master pulling the strings of your reproductive system, controlling your menstrual cycle, prepping your body for potential pregnancies, and even playing a role in your mood regulation.

However, during perimenopause, the years of heavy lifting start to take a toll, and estrogen begins to pack her bags, ready to leave for a long sabbatical. As a result, your body shifts from its reproductive phase into a new stage of life. But don't worry - this isn't a tragic goodbye. It's more like a fond farewell tour, with some rather memorable 'encore' moments (like those hot flashes and mood swings).

Estrogen has been the lead singer of your reproductive years, and as she steps back from the mic, the band plays on, adjusting to a new rhythm. It's a reminder that, as much as we'd like it, life doesn't come with auto-tune. But don't worry, you've got front-row seats, and we're here to help you understand every note.

SIGNS AND SYMPTOMS OF PERIMENOPAUSE

Roller coasters can be fun, right? The thrill, the unexpected turns, the heart-pounding adrenaline rush. But imagine being on one without knowing when the next drop or twist is coming. That's a bit of what perimenopause feels like, a hormonal roller coaster.

This phase, akin to the hormonal equivalent of a Jackson Pollock painting, is characterized by an assortment of signs and symptoms. Your body, your emotions, and even your sleep might seem like they're playing a strange game of charades that you didn't sign up for. In this section, we're going to decode the signs, uncover the symptoms, and, most importantly, reassure you that you're not alone in this ride.

Just remember, everyone's perimenopause journey is unique - some might experience these symptoms in spades, and others might just get a sprinkle. The key is to understand what's happening, so you can better navigate the unpredictable waves. Now, let's dive in and face these symptoms head-on.

Irregular Periods

Now, imagine this. Your menstrual cycle, for the longest time, has been like your reliable old sedan, purring along with minimal hiccups. But suddenly, it's more like a moody sports car, vrooming when you least expect it and stalling when you most need it. Welcome to the era of irregular periods, courtesy of perimenopause.

Irregular periods are one of the most telltale signs of peri-menopause. These can range from very light to extremely heavy and can last anywhere from two to seven days or longer. You might even have your period twice in one month or not at all for several months. It's like your hormones decided to throw a rave party and forgot to send you the memo.

In early perimenopause, you might notice your periods getting closer together, maybe every 24 to 26 days, especially if your cycle was always a bit shorter. Think of this phase as the appe-tizer, a little taste of what's to come. On the other hand, late perimenopause is the main course, where you may go two to three months without menstruating at all. However, don't ring the menopause bell just yet. You only officially reach menopause after a full year without periods.

Hot Flashes and Sleep Problems

Perimenopause, unfortunately, comes with its share of drama, starring hot flashes and sleep problems. Hot flashes, also known as vasomotor symptoms, are like mini internal heat waves. You can be calmly sipping your morning coffee, and suddenly you feel like you've been teleported to the Sahara.

The heart races, the face flushes, and you are the unwilling host of your very own tropical island party.

Now, if you were planning on escaping these hot flashes in the cool tranquility of sleep, I have some news for you. Perimenopause can cause disruptions to your sleep, too. Imagine you've just found the perfect sleeping position, the pillow is at the right angle, and the room is dark, and bam! You're wide awake. That's perimenopause playing tricks on your sleep.

Mood Changes

Entering the perimenopause stage might make you feel like you're on an emotional roller coaster. One moment you're laughing at a meme, and the next, you're crying because your favorite character in a TV show spilled their coffee. Mood changes, my friend, are an integral part of the perimenopause package.

These mood swings can often be attributed to hormonal fluctuations. It's a bit like having teenagers in the house. You never quite know what you're going to get. Estrogen, which was once your steady companion, is now fluctuating, leading to increased irritability, sudden bouts of sadness, and even depression in some cases. But worry not, understanding these changes can help you manage them better, and before you know it, you'll be cruising through perimenopause like a pro.

Vaginal and Bladder Problems

Remember that once-reliable car we talked about earlier? The one that's now playing tricks on you? Well, it turns out, it doesn't just stop at periods. The fluctuating estrogen levels during perimenopause can also play a role in vaginal and bladder health.

Decreased estrogen can lead to the thinning and drying of vaginal tissues, resulting in what's scientifically known as "vaginal atrophy," but let's call it "the Sahara syndrome." It can lead to discomfort during sexual activity and increased susceptibility to urinary and vaginal infections. You might also experience urinary incontinence, that uninvited guest that shows up when you laugh, cough, or even exercise. It's like a surprise party nobody asked for. But remember, there are treatments available, and it's important to discuss these changes with your healthcare provider and track the changes you experience, whether you think they are related or unrelated to perimenopause.

Decreasing Fertility

When it comes to fertility during perimenopause, the situation gets a little tricky. As you sail into the perimenopausal seas, your ovaries start acting like a moody artist, sometimes producing eggs, sometimes not. The result? A decrease in fertility.

During perimenopause, the irregularity in ovulation makes conception more challenging but not impossible. So, if you're not interested in adding a new member to your family, make sure you're still employing some form of birth control until you reach menopause. It's like a last call at a bar; there may be limited options, but there's still potential.

Changes in Sexual Function

Ah, the topic nobody wants to talk about, but everyone wants to know about: sexual function during perimenopause. As estrogen levels take a nosedive, so too can your sexual desire. Also, the changes in vaginal tissue we mentioned earlier can lead to discomfort during sex.

Think of it as an unfortunate game of dominos, where one tile of the hormonal balance topples, triggering a chain of events. Lower estrogen can lead to decreased libido and changes in sexual comfort. But fear not, just as you can pick up and reorder dominos, there are treatments, products, and supplements that can help restore your sexual function. As always, communicating these changes with your partner and healthcare provider can lead to effective solutions.

Loss of Bone

Now, let's talk about your bones, your body's structural pillars. During perimenopause, the reduction in estrogen levels can cause some interference in the bone-building business. The process of bone remodeling, where old bone is replaced with new, might be disrupted.

It's like having a construction crew (your bone cells) that's been consistently working on a site (your bones), but suddenly, some of their equipment (estrogen) starts disappearing. The result is that the demolition part of the crew (osteoclasts) starts working overtime, and the building part (osteoblasts) can't keep up. The result? A risk of osteoporosis. But don't worry, it's not all doom and gloom. With the right lifestyle adjustments and medical interventions, you can keep your skeleton sturdy and healthy.

Changing Cholesterol Levels

Just when you thought perimenopause had thrown all it could at you, it shows up with a curveball - changing cholesterol levels. It's like your body's lipids decided to play a game of seesaw. Low-density lipoprotein (LDL), often labeled as 'bad cholesterol,' can creep up, while high-density lipoprotein (HDL), the 'good cholesterol,' might decide to take a dip.

These changes are just another example of how fluctuating hormones can rock the boat in unexpected ways. But remember, knowing is half the battle. Regular check-ups and maintaining a balanced diet and lifestyle can help you manage these shifts and keep your lipid levels in a harmonious balance.

WHEN TO SEE A DOCTOR

You wouldn't try to fix a spaceship with duct tape and a hammer, right? Well, consider your body the spaceship and a doctor the qualified, NASA-trained engineer. Sometimes, despite our best efforts to self-diagnose and self-treat, we need to turn to the professionals. Navigating the twists and turns of perimenopause can sometimes leave us feeling lost in space, and that's when we need to find the right person to guide us back home. In this section, we'll discuss when to see a doctor and why it's crucial not to take this journey alone.

Importance of Seeking Medical Attention

In our era of instant gratification, Google has become the new-age oracle for all our queries. From "Why does my cat stare at me?" to "is it normal to forget where I left my keys five times a day?" – we tend to rely heavily on our digital doctor. But when it comes to perimenopause, Dr. Google might not be enough.

Seeking medical attention is like hiring a professional guide while hiking up a challenging trail. They know the route, the tricky turns, and how to avoid the nasty poison ivy. Health professionals can give you personalized advice based on your medical history, current symptoms, and future health goals. They're your trusty sidekick through this unpredictable adventure, ensuring you don't end up fighting the bad guys alone, but the trick is finding the right Robin for your Batman.

Here are a few reasons why you should consider seeing a doctor:

1. **Customized Care:** No two bodies are the same, and hence, the journey through perimenopause is also unique for each individual. A healthcare professional can provide personalized care and advice that suits your specific needs and situation and help you identify what symptoms are perimenopause associated and which are not.

2. **Early Detection:** Regular check-ups can help detect any serious conditions or complications at an early stage. The sooner the diagnosis, the better the chances of effective management and treatment.

3. **Medical Therapies:** If you're experiencing severe symptoms, a healthcare professional can guide you about possible medical interventions. This can range from hormonal therapies to lifestyle modification strategies.

Symptoms that Warrant a Doctor's Visit

If you start to notice that your perimenopause symptoms are taking the wheel and dictating how you live your daily life, it might be time to see a doctor. Also, keep in mind that although some symptoms are common during this phase, others might not be related to perimenopause and could indicate a different health issue.

Think of it like this: your car's check engine light is on, it's making a strange noise, and the brakes are feeling a bit spongy. Sure, you could ignore it all and hope for the best, or you could take it to a mechanic to get it sorted.

Here's a checklist of symptoms that should prompt you to schedule an appointment:

1. **Heavy or Prolonged Periods:** If the "monthly guest" decides to overstay her welcome or arrives with a piece of unusually heavy luggage, it's time to seek medical advice.
2. **Severe Hot Flashes:** If your internal thermostat seems to be out of control, leading to discomfort and disrupted sleep, a healthcare professional can help manage this.
3. **Mood Swings:** Emotional rollercoasters can be hard to handle. If you find drastic mood changes impacting your quality of life, it might be time to seek help.
4. **Unexpected Weight Gain:** If the scale seems to be creeping up despite your best efforts, it might be worth discussing with a doctor.

Remember, there's no heroism in suffering in silence. Seeking help and advice when you need it is the best thing you can do for your health and happiness. You're not alone on this crime-fighting adventure through perimenopause – don't hesitate to ask for the guidance you need to lean on Robin.

Finding the Right Doctor

If menopause is a crime-fighting adventure, then consider the doctor your Robin. While it's vital to listen to your body, having a knowledgeable and compassionate professional on your side is equally important. Your body is like a complex, intricate machine, and understanding its subtle changes and signs can be daunting. This is where a doctor, your guide, your Robin in this journey comes into play.

However, finding the right doctor is not always a straightforward task. My personal journey through menopause taught me that the hard way. Despite consulting with numerous doctors, most of them dismissed my concerns as "just going through menopause". It took me seven tries to find my Robin, a doctor who viewed my issues as important, gave me a variety of options, and explained the process. The dismissal I, and so many women, experience, is a reflection of a broader issue: there is a significant gap in medical training when it comes to menopause.

A 2018 study published in *Menopause Review* found that over 80% of surveyed medical students and doctors considered their knowledge of menopause to be insufficient. This lack of training is not just confined to one country or region; it's a global issue. Consequently, many women are left feeling unheard, dismissed, and misunderstood.

So, how do you find a doctor who not only understands the nuances of menopause but also listens and empathizes with your experience?

The answer lies in persistence and advocacy. Don't settle for the first doctor you see if they don't acknowledge your concerns. Shop around for healthcare the way you would for a car or a house. Do your research, ask for referrals, read reviews, and always trust your instincts; when you meet your sidekick, you will know. It's your body, your health, and your journey - you have the right to be heard, understood, and respected.

When you finally find a doctor who ticks all these boxes, you'll feel a sense of relief and validation. Remember, you're not just "going through menopause"; you're navigating a significant life change, and you deserve a healthcare provider who recognizes that.

Your voice matters. Your health matters. And finding the right doctor is the first step towards a smoother, more informed journey through menopause.

CAUSES AND RISK FACTORS

Remember those teen years when your hormones decided to host a non-stop rave inside your body? Well, think of perimenopause as the "one last hurrah" for these hormonal party-goers before they retire. Perimenopause is essentially a roller-coaster ride of hormonal changes, and understanding these changes can help us grasp why we experience certain symptoms. In this section, we'll take a journey through the wild world of hormones and their role in perimenopause and explore why some of us might face this transitional period earlier than others.

The Role of Estrogen and Progesterone

Estrogen and progesterone are the headliners of the hormonal gig that is perimenopause. They've been your faithful sidekicks since puberty, involved in everything from regulating your periods to preparing your body for pregnancy. But as you approach menopause, these hormonal besties decide to go a bit rogue.

Imagine estrogen as that over-enthusiastic friend who's always switching the party location. One minute, it's up high; the next, it's down low. This unpredictable fluctuation is what leads to the many symptoms of perimenopause. And progesterone? Well, it's like that friend who promised to come to the party but ends up flaking out more often, especially when the ovaries stop releasing eggs.

So, you see, perimenopause is pretty much a hormone fest with both your hormonal friends acting out of character. But fear not; understanding their quirks can help us handle them better.

Early Onset of Perimenopause

Most of us expect to deal with perimenopause in our 40s or even later, but what about when it comes knocking a bit early? Like that cousin who shows up at Thanksgiving dinner a week ahead of time, early onset perimenopause can catch us off-guard. There are several factors that might lead to this early arrival, so let's uncover them:

1. **Smoking:** Our puffs of pleasure might seem harmless in our youth, but cigarettes are essentially time machines that fast-forward us to menopause. The toxic chemicals in cigarettes affect how our body produces estrogen, pushing us into the perimenopause phase earlier than non-smokers. So, if you're lighting up, you're essentially inviting perimenopause to the party ahead of time.

2. **Family History:** Our family passes down many things: grandma's secret apple pie recipe, dad's oddly shaped toes, and, perhaps, early perimenopause. If the women in your family have a history of early menopause, you might also be more likely to hear the perimenopausal knock on your door sooner.

3. **Cancer Treatment:** Cancer treatments like chemotherapy and radiation therapy are like a storm for the ovaries. They can cause damage that leads to the early onset of perimenopause. It's one of those uninvited side effects that no one really wants, but preparing for it can make the journey smoother.

4. **Hysterectomy:** Hysterectomy, a surgery to remove the uterus, is like unplugging the DJ at the hormonal gig. While you might still have your ovaries (the

estrogen producers), the lack of a uterus changes the hormonal dynamics, often leading to early perimenopause.

Understanding the causes and risk factors of perimenopause can help us better navigate this journey. It reminds us that perimenopause is not some random event but a complex interplay of our hormones, lifestyle choices, genetics, and, sometimes, medical treatments. The more aware we are, the better prepared we can be. Because knowledge, as they say, is power. Or, in this case, the right kind of hormonal power!

DEALING WITH PERIMENOPAUSE: ACTIONABLE STEPS

If perimenopause is an uninvited house guest, then think of this section as your eviction guide. Although you can't exactly kick perimenopause out (it does have squatter's rights, after all), there are ways to manage it so that it doesn't rule your roost. We've got a smorgasbord of practical steps for you, from dietary hacks to healing practices from the East and even a tour of medical treatments. Strap in and get ready to take some notes!

Diet and Exercise Changes

Let's start with some food for thought—literally. As it turns out, perimenopause is one of those picky eaters. It tends to make a fuss when you're chowing down on processed foods or overindulging in that bottle of Cabernet. The good news is, it's actually a fan of whole foods and hydration, so think lean proteins, fruits, veggies, and yes, water! Load up on calcium and vitamin D, too. They're like the superhero duo for your bone health. And remember, portion control is key, even when it comes to the good stuff.

Moving on to exercise, think of it as the house party that keeps perimenopause's wild behavior in check. Regular activity is like a lullaby for your chaotic hormones, helping to reduce hot flashes and improve sleep. Cardio is great, but it also includes strength training and flexibility exercises in your routine. They'll help keep your bones strong and your joints limber— after all, who doesn't like a flexible guest?

Non-Western Healing Practices

Now, we're heading east! No, we're not planning an exotic vacation (though that sounds delightful!). We're exploring healing practices from other parts of the world. We're talking about yoga, acupuncture, and meditation. These techniques can help you keep your zen amidst the perimenopause storm.

Yoga, for example, is not just about turning your body into a human pretzel. The right poses can help manage hot flashes and mood swings. Meditation, on the other hand, is like a tranquility workshop for your mind, perfect for combating anxiety and sleep issues. And acupuncture? Well, it's not everyone's cup of tea, but some women swear by its hormone-balancing effects.

Medical Treatments

If you're still feeling the heat of perimenopause, don't fret. It might be time to knock on your doctor's door for some medical treatments. The medical community has an arsenal of solutions, from hormone therapy to certain antidepressants. And they're not just pulling these out of a magician's hat; these treatments are backed by extensive research and can be tailored to your unique needs.

Hormone therapy is a bit like a celebrity impersonator at the hormonal gig, mimicking the actions of estrogen and progesterone to ease perimenopause symptoms. Then there are low-dose antidepressants, which may sound drastic but are actually quite helpful in managing hot flashes. Plus, if you're dealing with vaginal dryness (an uncharming parting gift from perimenopause), there are topical treatments available, such as creams, gels, or tablets, that are applied or inserted directly into the vagina to provide localized relief.

Remember, reaching out for medical help is not an admission of defeat; it's a proactive step toward reclaiming your well-being. So, if you've tried all the kale salads and downward dogs you can stomach and are still struggling, it's time to connect with a healthcare professional.

In the end, dealing with perimenopause is about finding the right balance that works for you. It's about trying, adjusting, and sometimes trying again. But armed with these actionable steps, you're well on your way to making your journey through perimenopause a lot smoother. Because let's be real: it might be an uninvited guest, but that doesn't mean it gets to throw the party.

THE PERIMENOPAUSE LIFESTYLE ASSESSMENT QUIZ

Who doesn't love a good quiz? Especially one that's all about you! This isn't your standard pub quiz or the dreaded pop quiz from high school. No, this is a choose-your-own-adventure of sorts. A lifestyle assessment quiz designed to help you better understand your perimenopausal journey. Are you ready? Let's dive in!

How would you rate your physical activity level?

A. Sedentary: My idea of an extreme sport is a Netflix marathon.

B. Lightly Active: I'll take the stairs instead of the elevator, thank you very much.

C. Moderately Active: I've got my gym membership, and I'm not afraid to use it!

D. Very Active: I sweat more than a hot flash at an aerobic dance class.

How would you describe your diet?

A. Fast Food Fanatic: If it comes with fries, I'm game.

B. Moderation Maven: I indulge but try to balance it out with some fruits and veggies.

C. Health Conscious: Quinoa salad and kale smoothies are my jam.

D. Clean Eating Champion: I haven't met a whole food I didn't like.

How often do you experience high levels of stress?

A. Always: My life is a reality TV show level of drama.

B. Often: Work, kids, life...it's a juggling act.

C. Sometimes: I've got my stressors, but I take time to decompress.

D. Rarely: I've found my zen, and nothing can shake it.

How would you rate your sleep quality?

A. Poor: I spend more time counting sheep than I'd like to admit.

B. Fair: I get by, but those 8 hours are elusive.

C. Good: I'm out as soon as my head hits the pillow.

D. Excellent: I sleep like a baby and wake up refreshed.

How would you rate your emotional well-being?

A. Struggling: I feel like I'm riding a rollercoaster of emotions.

B. Coping: It's a challenge, but I'm hanging in there.

C. Balanced: I have my ups and downs, but I feel in control.

D. Thriving: I'm as happy as a clam at high tide.

Remember, this quiz isn't a diagnosis tool. It's just a snapshot of your lifestyle during perimenopause. Each answer provides a clue to what might help you navigate this phase more comfortably. If you're a lot of As and Bs, maybe it's time to look at making some changes. If you're scoring Cs and Ds, you're probably already doing a great job handling the perimenopause waves. Either way, use this quiz as a tool to help guide your journey and remember, the perimenopause monster isn't invincible, and neither are you. You've got this!

STORY TIME: MARIA'S JOURNEY THROUGH PERIMENOPAUSE

Maria is a 48-year-old high school history teacher who could probably recite the dates of every significant battle in the last three centuries. She's a mother of two teenagers, owner of a feisty Corgi named 'Churchill,' and a world-class salsa dancer in her living room. Maria is no stranger to life's ups and downs, but when she started experiencing what she later recognized as perimenopause symptoms, even her vast historical knowledge couldn't provide the answers she needed.

Her perimenopausal journey started subtly, sneakily. Picture a ninja tiptoeing into a silent room, leaving no trace of its presence. Maria's periods, as punctual as a Swiss watch, began to go 'freestyle.' Her sleep, previously like a log in the quiet forest, started to resemble a series of catnaps. Hot flashes? Oh, they arrived like uninvited guests at a dinner party, turning Maria's body into a furnace.

However, Maria, being the warrior she is, didn't let these 'hormonal hiccups' phase her. As a single mother of two lively teenagers, she continued her passionate history lectures, kept dancing in her living room, and yes, managed the teenage drama at home. But the real test was yet to come.

This was when Maria's subtle symptoms turned into a 'perfect storm.' The irregular periods became more unpredictable, and the hot flashes intensified, playing havoc with her sleep, which was now more like an elusive butterfly. She experienced mood swings as volatile as the stock market on a bad day. Even her passion for salsa seemed to fade a bit. And her students started noticing 'Ms. History Buff' was losing her mojo.

But Maria, undeterred, took the bull by the horns. She sought medical advice, started a dialogue with her friends experiencing the same changes, and educated herself on perimenopause. She started incorporating healthier foods into her diet, walking Churchill more often, and practicing mindfulness to manage stress. She even turned to acupuncture and found it surprisingly helpful in managing hot flashes.

Fast forward to the present day, Maria is still riding the perimenopause wave. She has her good days when she feels like a rock star and others when she's more akin to a washed-up one-hit wonder. But she's armed with knowledge, coping mechanisms, and a support system, making her journey through perimenopause not just bearable but even empowering at times.

And guess what? She's even started a 'Perimenopause Support Club' at her school for other staff navigating the same tumultuous seas, becoming the captain of the ship she once felt adrift in.

The moral of Maria's story? Perimenopause might seem like a hormonal tsunami at first, but with the right tools, information, and attitude, it's navigable. And as Maria would say, "It's not about the storm, but how you dance in the rain... or, in my case, salsa!"

So keep dancing, my friends. Maria sure is.

KEY TAKEAWAYS

1. Perimenopause is a transition phase marked by hormonal changes and varied symptoms.
2. Symptoms range from irregular periods and hot flashes to mood changes.
3. Lifestyle changes, medical treatments, and alternative practices can manage symptoms.
4. Early symptom recognition and medical advice ensure effective management.
5. Embracing this phase with knowledge and self-care can be empowering.

FINAL THOUGHTS

Perimenopause is as unpredictable as a British summer, and yet, it's a journey that every woman aboard the ship of life must embark on. But remember, dear readers, that while the waves of hormonal changes may seem daunting, you're not just a passenger on this voyage. You're the captain, fully capable of steering your ship through the choppy waters towards calmer seas.

In this chapter, we've journeyed through the twists and turns of perimenopause, from understanding its biology, recognizing its symptoms, exploring its causes, to seeking medical advice, and finally managing it with a variety of approaches (more specifics to come). We've also shared a few laughs because why not?

The essence here isn't just to survive perimenopause but to conquer it - to dance in the rain (or the hormonal storm), just like our perimenopausal pioneer Maria. Remember, no phase of life, not even perimenopause, can rob you of your vitality and spirit. You got this!

As we close this chapter, let's remember that science still has a lot to explore in this realm. It's a journey, much like the perimenopause itself. Speaking of science, brace yourself as our next chapter delves deeper into 'The Science of Menopause: The Knowns and the Unknowns.' Stay tuned!

THE SCIENCE OF MENOPAUSE: THE KNOWNS AND THE UNKNOWNS

Menopause is like puberty's final exam, and life didn't even provide a study guide. One day, your body is running smoothly like a well-oiled machine, and the next, it seems like someone hit all the buttons on your hormonal elevator. Up, down, and all around, you're in for a ride, my friend. But fear not! You are not alone, and no, you are not malfunctioning.

Menopause, often seen as a bewildering phase, is truly the mark of a seasoned life. Just as wine matures and develops complexity over time, so do we, right? Though some may perceive this as a period of loss, I invite you to view it as a celebration of evolution.

In this chapter, we're diving deep into the waters of menopause. Not just dipping our toes in, we're doing a full-on cannonball. We'll talk about the essence of menopause, its role, its impact, and why it isn't just an annoying period at the end of your sentence. Get it? "Period." But let's keep the menstrual puns at bay for now.

We'll delve into what happens when the body decides to shut down the fertility factory. But I promise, it's not all hot flashes and mood swings. There's much more to it. This is not just a transformation; it's a rite of passage, a transcendence to a new sphere of life.

Remember, this isn't some dusty, old biology textbook. So, expect a lively discussion filled with facts, personal stories, and even a sprinkle of humor to lighten the mood. After all, life's too short to be serious all the time. So buckle up, we're heading straight into the eye of the menopause storm. And who knows? We might even find a rainbow on the other side.

UNMASKING MENOPAUSE

We've all heard of menopause. It's that period in a woman's life (pardon the pun), typically between 45 and 55 years of age, when menstruation says adieu, and the ovaries put up the 'closed for business' sign. But let's unpack it a bit more.

Simply put, menopause is the end of a woman's menstrual cycle. It's officially diagnosed after a woman has gone 12 months without a menstrual period. But ladies, if you think this is all about you, I hate to break it to you, it's not. It's a family affair. Husbands, children, friends – everyone's invited to the party! In fact, menopause can be such a life-altering experience that the whole neighborhood might feel the heat, literally and figuratively!

Now, while the definition of menopause seems straightforward enough, there's much more going on beneath the surface. This is not just about periods going AWOL; it's about a shift in hormone production that can lead to a medley of symptoms. It's like your body throwing a hormonal rave without asking for your permission.

The Concept of Menopause: A Biopsychosocial Perspective

Okay, it's time to put on your thinking caps. Let's talk about menopause from a biopsychosocial perspective. Don't let that hefty term intimidate you; it just means we're considering biological, psychological, and social aspects. It's like the trifecta of menopause understanding!

Biologically, menopause is the cessation of ovulation and a decrease in the production of hormones, mainly estrogen and progesterone.

Psychologically, menopause can lead to mood swings, irritability, and sometimes, feelings akin to teenage angst. So, if you suddenly have the urge to paint your room black and blast heavy metal music, don't panic; it's just your hormones playing DJ.

From a social perspective, menopause is often seen as a marker of aging, which can carry a negative connotation. However, with a shift in mindset, it can be viewed as a transition into a new, liberated phase of life, free from the worry of unplanned pregnancies. So, while the biological symptoms might be unavoidable, the psychological and social experiences of menopause are pretty subjective.

Brief Historical Perspective of Menopause

Let's step into the time machine and look back at how the understanding and perception of menopause have evolved over the years.

Back in the day, menopause was often shrouded in mystery, with not much known about its cause or symptoms. It was like the 'He Who Must Not Be Named' of women's health. There were times when women experiencing menopausal symptoms were thought to be 'hysterical' or 'possessed.' Fast forward to today, and we've come a long way, with a plethora of research now available on the subject.

Menopause has had quite a journey, from being a taboo topic whispered only in hushed tones to being discussed openly in books, on talk shows, and all over the internet. We've gone from seeing it as a sign of aging and decline to recognizing it as a natural transition, a testament to a woman's strength and resilience. This change in perspective hasn't come easy, though. It's the result of tireless efforts by women's health advocates, healthcare professionals, and fearless women who refused to suffer in silence.

So, while the hormonal dance of menopause might still be a rollercoaster ride, remember, you're not riding it alone. Our understanding and acceptance of menopause have grown, making this journey a bit easier to navigate for all women. Menopause is not an ending; it's a beginning, the dawn of a new phase filled with opportunities and growth.

RELATIONSHIP REVAMP: MENOPAUSE'S UNEXPECTED GUEST

Menopause might be a personal journey, but it doesn't travel solo. It brings along an uninvited guest to our relationships, creating a ripple effect that reaches far beyond the person experiencing it. And just like a new roommate moving in, it demands adjustments, patience, and heaps of understanding from everyone involved.

Relationship with Self: The Inner Tumult

Menopause is a bit like an unexpected houseguest - it shows up unannounced and proceeds to rearrange your furniture. And when that furniture includes everything from your physical appearance to your emotional stability, the results can be...interesting, to say the least.

As estrogen levels take a nosedive, you might find your self-confidence sliding down that slope with them. Suddenly, you're playing host to a barrage of new experiences: hot flashes that make you feel like a human volcano, mood swings that could rival a pendulum on steroids, and night sweats that leave you contemplating the feasibility of nocturnal showers.

And then there are the physical changes. Who needs the unpredictability of a thrilling suspense novel when you've got the drama of menopausal weight gain and sagging skin? It's as if your body has suddenly decided to become an artist, and its chosen medium is your waistline and skin elasticity.

A 2009 study published in the journal *Maturitas* highlights how menopausal symptoms, particularly hot flashes, insomnia, and depression, can negatively impact a woman's quality of life and self-esteem. But remember, it's essential to extend kindness and understanding to oneself during this time. Think of it as getting to know a new version of yourself - like meeting a long-lost twin who just happens to have a flair for the dramatic.

Personal Relationships: The Emotional Quake

When it comes to personal relationships, menopause might as well be a bull in a china shop. It's not subtle, it's not gentle, and it can leave you and your partner feeling like you're constantly on clean-up duty.

From a dip in libido that can turn your once-fiery passion into the faint flicker of a dying candle to painful sex due to vaginal dryness that makes the Sahara seem wet by comparison, menopause can throw quite the wrench in your love life. And then there are the mood swings that leave partners unsure if they're dealing with Dr. Jekyll or Mrs. Hyde.

But as any good relationship counselor will tell you, communication is key. A 2018 review in *The Journal of Women's Health* highlighted how menopause can significantly impact a woman's sexual function and relationship with her partner, but it also stressed the importance of open communication and mutual understanding. Menopause is not a solo journey; it's a shared experience that can strengthen a couple's bond if navigated with patience and love.

Social Relationships: The Invisible Tsunami

Imagine being on a merry-go-round, but instead of colorful horses and cheerful music, you've got hot flashes, sleep disturbances, and inexplicable mood swings. Welcome to menopause. Such symptoms can transform even the most delightful social engagement into an exhausting chore.

Your friends may not understand why you've suddenly lost interest in your regular book club meetings or why you've turned into an irritable version of the woman they've known for years.

And can you blame them? Menopause is often shrouded in mystery, a taboo topic whispered behind closed doors. But opening up the conversation can pave the way for better understanding and support. After all, if we can openly discuss broken bones and flu shots, why not hot flashes and night sweats? A study in Menopause Review points to the social stigma associated with menopause, urging societies to lift the veil of silence surrounding it.

Menopause is an unexpected guest that reshapes our lives and relationships in ways we never imagined. But by bringing the conversation out of the shadows and fostering understanding, we can make this phase less about surviving and more about thriving.

THE KNOWNS: CURRENT UNDERSTANDING OF MENOPAUSE

Now, let's dive into the know-hows of menopause. Imagine it as a Pandora's box of "What's happening to my body?" But don't worry, unlike Pandora's version, this box contains knowledge and insights that make menopause less of a monster and more of a, well, let's say, an uninvited house guest who eventually becomes a part of the family.

The Nitty-Gritty of Menopause: The Biological Process

The curtain rises on menopause, not with a magician's flourish, but through an intricate, gradual biological process. The protagonists of this tale are your ovaries. Beyond their famed egg-production role, ovaries are like diligent factory workers, tirelessly synthesizing hormones, namely estrogen and progesterone. From orchestrating the menstrual cycle to preserving bone health, these hormones are essential cogs in the machinery of the female body.

The onset of menopause isn't a meticulously timed event. Rather, it loosely corresponds to a timeline, typically between the ages of 45 and 55. Picture it as an unexpected, though not unwelcome, visitor who might drop by anytime during a decade-long window.

As the biological clock ticks away, your ovaries begin to hang their "out of service" signs. In turn, the production of estrogen and progesterone gradually tapers off, akin to the retirement of an efficient CEO, leaving the body to adapt to a new era of management.

Estrogen: The Puppeteer of Bodily Functions

When it comes to the multitude of roles estrogen plays in the body, one can't help but marvel. The functions of this powerful hormone extend well beyond regulating your menstrual cycle. Estrogen is instrumental in a wide array of bodily functions, from ensuring healthy skin to safeguarding cardiovascular health and even influencing mood and cognitive function.

One might liken estrogen to a skilled conductor, orchestrating the harmony of bodily functions with precision. Its influence is so pervasive that even slight changes in its levels can throw the whole symphony off balance.

With the onset of menopause, estrogen levels start to decline, leaving the body to grapple with new, uncharted terrain. To continue the conductor metaphor, it's as though the main maestro has left the stage, and the orchestra needs to learn how to keep the music playing.

During this transition, a variety of symptoms may emerge. These are manifestations of the body's attempts to adjust to fluctuating estrogen levels, just as a finely-tuned instrument responds to changes in atmospheric pressure or temperature. Understanding the complex symphony of estrogen can provide valuable insights into the whys and hows of these menopause-related changes, making it easier to navigate this crucial period of a woman's life.

Putting Menopause Under the Microscope: The NICE Approach to Diagnosis

Getting to the heart of menopause isn't a walk in the park. It's not like there's a big red button that lights up when menopause begins. But don't fret; science has a method to this madness. Let's talk about the detective work involved in diagnosing menopause, guided by the National Institute for Health and Care Excellence (NICE).

To begin with, doctors play something of a game of "Clue," piecing together evidence to deduce whether a woman is menopausal. It's not as glamorous as Miss Scarlet in the billiard room with the candlestick, but it's critical nonetheless.

According to the NICE guidelines, the key players in this medical mystery are age and menstrual irregularities. Menopause usually comes knocking between the ages of 45 and 55. If a woman in this age bracket experiences irregular periods or no periods for about 12 months, the suspicion is raised. But hold on; it's not time to declare 'case closed' just yet.

For women under 45 who exhibit these symptoms, more detective work may be needed. Doctors may recommend a blood test to measure hormone levels. This test typically checks the level of follicle-stimulating hormone (FSH), which rises during menopause. However, hormone levels can fluctuate significantly, and a single test might not give a definitive answer. So, it's a bit like tracking a moving target.

Moreover, diagnosing menopause in women who use hormonal contraception is more complex since these treatments can mask menopausal symptoms. It's like trying to solve a mystery while the usual suspects have a solid alibi.

To clarify this scenario, NICE provides specific guidelines. They suggest stopping hormonal contraception and waiting for at least two menstrual cycles before measuring FSH levels. It might sound like a bit of a waiting game, but it's crucial for ensuring an accurate diagnosis.

Once the diagnosis of menopause is confirmed, the next step is managing its effects - a saga that merits its own discussion and one we will have in the upcoming chapters. Remember, menopause isn't just a series of biological events. It's a journey, with every woman taking a slightly different path. The diagnosis is just the beginning; there's a whole lot more to this adventure.

THE UNKNOWNS: WHAT SCIENCE STILL DOESN'T UNDERSTAND

You've got to love how even with all our advances in medical science, there's still an element of mystery. It's like we're living in a Sherlock Holmes novel, with menopause playing the role of the elusive culprit. There are still aspects of menopause that are as mysterious as the depths of the ocean. Let's unravel some of these riddles, shall we?

The Purpose of Menopause

"Why do we even go through menopause?" you might ask. Good question. And the answer is... we're not exactly sure. Sure, we understand the mechanics of it, but why it happens in the first place, why women outlive their reproductive years, is something of an evolutionary enigma.

The evolution of menopause remains an enigma. Like a compelling murder mystery, it's the 'why' that keeps scientists scratching their heads, not the 'how.' On a physiological level, we're clear: the ovaries cease releasing eggs, causing a decline in hormone production. But why, from an evolutionary stand-point, would women stop being able to reproduce midway through life?

Enter the "Grandmother Hypothesis," which has all the charm of a cozy mystery novel. The theory proposes that women cease to reproduce to help raise their grandchildren, thus ensuring the survival of their genes indirectly. It's a solid theory, but scientists are far from closing the case.

There's also the "Mother Hypothesis," arguing that as the risks of childbirth and childrearing increase with age, menopause protects older women from these risks. So, is it the nurturing grandma or the self-preserving mom? Or perhaps a story yet untold? Much like Agatha Christie's best works, the plot keeps thickening.

Determinants of the Functional Lifespan of Ovaries

Our ovaries, unfortunately, don't come with an expiration date. The transition to menopause typically starts between the ages of 45 and 55, but why is there such a broad range? What causes the ticking ovarian time bomb to finally go off?

Numerous factors likely come into play, from genetic variations to environmental influences. Some studies suggest a correlation between the age at which a woman's mother experienced menopause and her own menopausal timing, hinting at a genetic component. Other research indicates that lifestyle factors such as smoking can expedite the process. Still, this is akin to the 'chicken or the egg' conundrum – there are theories aplenty but no definitive answers yet.

Hormonal Fluctuations and their Effects on Bodily Functions

If menopause is a roller coaster, hormonal fluctuations are those adrenaline-inducing twists and turns. Declining estrogen levels can influence everything from your heart health to your memory. It's like trying to navigate through a funhouse mirror maze – disorienting and unpredictable.

Estrogen does more than just regulate menstruation; it's involved in cholesterol regulation, maintaining bone density, and even brain functions. So when its levels drop, the effects are felt body-wide. But how these hormonal changes translate into symptoms is a vastly complex process, and it's still not entirely understood. Like a cryptic crossword puzzle, we've only filled in some of the squares.

Individual Differences in Reaction to Changes in Estrogen Levels

The story of menopause is as unique as the woman who tells it. For some, the transition is a tempest, filled with hot flashes and night sweats. For others, it's a mild breeze, barely noticeable. But why such variation?

Factors such as genetics, lifestyle, and overall health likely play a part. Certain genetic variations, for example, have been associated with early-onset menopause. Lifestyle factors like diet and exercise, as well as underlying health conditions, can also influence the experience of menopause. But much like why some people can stomach the spiciest of peppers while others blanch at a hint of jalapeno, there's still much to learn about these individual differences. Just another layer of intrigue in the ongoing saga of menopause.

So, there you have it, a brief journey through the winding alleys of what we still don't understand about menopause. It's a reminder that every woman's journey is unique, and there's no "normal" way to experience this life stage. But don't worry, just because there are some unknowns doesn't mean we're wandering around in the dark. Up next, we'll explore some myths about menopause that have been busted by science. Stay tuned!

CREATING YOUR PERSONAL MENOPAUSE JOURNEY MAP

Well, if you've ever wanted to map something more personal than your morning jog route, here's your chance! You see, menopause, like any great journey, should come with its own map. Not the kind with 'X marks the spot,' but a map that will help you navigate the turbulent seas of hormonal change and guide you towards calmer waters.

Keeping a Menopause Journey Map is like having your very own personal diary and weather forecast rolled into one. It allows you to track symptoms, note changes in your lifestyle and emotions, and draw connections you might not have seen otherwise. It's like having your own scientific lab where you are both the scientist and the subject.

Here's how to set about mapping your journey:

1. Set up the Basic Structure

Your Journey Map is as unique as you, but it helps to start with a basic structure. Think of it like setting up a calendar or planner. Designate spaces for daily, weekly, and monthly entries. Your daily entries could track your symptoms and feelings, while weekly and monthly entries could be more reflective, noting changes and trends over time.

As you set up this structure, ensure it's flexible. You might want to track different symptoms or experiences as your journey evolves. You could add additional categories like 'Sleep Quality' or 'Stress Levels'. Remember, this isn't a rigid spreadsheet - it's a living, breathing record of your experience. Your map should be a combination of standard elements (like dates and symptom trackers) and personalized elements (like lifestyle changes, emotional health, and moments of joy).

Consider keeping a space for progress notes. Here, you can write longer reflections on your journey – what's working, what's challenging, and what you're learning about yourself. This can be a valuable tool for reflection and growth.

So not the crafty type, me either, so to make this journey easier and more reflective, I've created your very own Menopause

Journey Map titled *"Menopause Makeover: A Guided Journal for Transformation."* Available on Amazon, this journal is more than just a tracking tool. It's a companion that walks with you through your menopause journey, providing spaces for tracking symptoms, jotting down notes, and reflecting on your progress. And the best part? You're not just writing in a journal, you're writing your story. So why not make it a part of your journey?

Check out the *Menopause Makeover: A Guided Journal for Transformation* today!

2. Track Symptoms and Experiences

It's time to play detective! Each day, note any physical symptoms you experience - hot flashes, night sweats, fatigue, you name it. This isn't just about noting the negatives, though. Also, jot down the good days, the times you felt energetic and vibrant.

On the other side, track the intensity of these symptoms. Consider creating a rating system from 1-5, with 1 being "barely noticeable" and 5 being "intensely discomforting". This will help you visualize trends over time. Also, keep an eye on the triggers. Maybe spicy food exacerbates hot flashes, or caffeine triggers insomnia. Noting these patterns can help you manage your symptoms more effectively.

Don't forget to include notes on your menstrual cycle too. Changes in regularity, flow, and accompanying symptoms can provide crucial insights into your menopause journey.

3. Note Lifestyle Changes and Their Impacts

Are you trying a new exercise routine? Have you made dietary changes or started a new meditation practice? Make a note of these changes and observe how they impact your symptoms and overall well-being.

Keep tabs on your lifestyle habits and modifications. You might be surprised to find that small changes, like adding more fiber to your diet or incorporating gentle yoga, have significant impacts. Furthermore, noting these impacts can help you build a lifestyle that supports your well-being during menopause.

Beyond physical wellness, remember to track changes in your social and mental wellness routines. Did spending time with friends lift your mood? Did a new book make you see things differently? These subtle shifts can play a significant role in your menopause journey.

4. Record Emotional Changes and Coping Strategies

Your emotions are as much a part of your menopause journey as your physical symptoms. Record your emotional ups and downs and note what helps you cope. Maybe it's a walk in the park, a call with a good friend, or a new hobby that keeps your mind engaged.

Emotions can be tricky to track, but you can make it easier by noting your general mood for the day or recording specific emotional events. Did a work presentation make you unusually anxious? Did a family gathering leave you feeling unexpectedly low? Observing these emotional responses can help you understand your emotional landscape during menopause better.

Remember, it's not just about recording the lows. Capture the highs, too - moments of joy, pride, or accomplishment. These can act as reminders that menopause, like any journey, is filled with peaks and valleys, and they all contribute to your unique experience.

5. Reflect on and Learn from Your Journey Map

Your Menopause Journey Map isn't just a log of events; it's a source of insight. Take time each week or month to look back, see patterns, and discover what works for you and what doesn't. Remember, knowledge is power - the more you understand about your menopause journey, the better equipped you'll be to navigate it.

Your map can be an invaluable tool for discussions with your healthcare provider. It can provide them with a detailed picture of your menopause experience, helping them tailor their advice and treatment to your unique journey.

Remember, your Menopause Journey Map is your personal tool - use it in a way that helps you best. Happy mapping!

STORY TIME: AMBER'S RECIPE FOR EMBRACING MENOPAUSE

Once upon a time, in a bustling city, we meet Amber, a 52-year-old chef, a food truck owner, and a woman on a mission. Amber has always lived her life in the fast lane. Always on the move and always taking on new adventures. However, in recent years, a different kind of adventure has begun to unfold – one she wasn't exactly prepared for.

It started quietly, with missed periods here and there. Initially, she attributed it to stress, dismissing it as nothing more than a temporary blip in her otherwise reliable monthly routine. But as months turned into a year, and the intervals between her periods stretched further apart, Amber started to wonder.

And then came the hot flashes, as unpredictable and dramatic as a celebrity chef's temper tantrum. They would hit her without warning, turning her into a walking, talking, profusely sweating volcano. The sudden surges of heat were bad enough during the winter months, but in the sweltering heat of the summer, they were unbearable.

Amber, who took pride in her boundless energy and vitality, was left puzzled and drained. She felt betrayed by her own body. Determined to find answers, she found herself venturing into various doctor's offices across the city. One, a dismissive older man who told her it was 'just women's troubles'. Another well-meaning woman who sympathized but offered little in the way of actionable advice.

Then, as hope was dwindling, Amber found herself walking into the office of Dr. Harper, a renowned gynecologist in the city. He listened, he understood, and most importantly, he offered her the advice she desperately needed. Most importantly, he finally labeled it for her; it's menopause.

The word "menopause" hung in the air between them, a strange mix of relief and trepidation. Relief because Amber finally had a name for her predicament, and trepidation because, well, she was entering uncharted waters. Dr. Harper provided Amber with a wealth of information, sparking her interest and prompting her to learn more about menopause.

Amber dove into the world of menopause with the same tenacity with which she mastered complex recipes. She learned about the hormonal symphony orchestrated by her body, the intricate dance of estrogen and progesterone, the grand divas of her reproductive system that were now taking their final bow.

Her understanding grew, as did her empathy for her own body. She saw menopause not as a malfunction but as a natural progression, a new stage of life. The transition wasn't easy; the physical discomfort, the mood swings, and the often dismissive societal attitudes were tough to handle. But she wasn't one to back down from a challenge.

Amber started to take better care of her body, incorporating healthier options into her diet, introducing gentle yoga into her routine, and practicing mindfulness to manage her stress levels. She also explored medical options, talking to her doctor about the pros and cons of hormone replacement therapy.

She began to share her journey openly with others, breaking the silence that often surrounds menopause. Amber's food truck, once only famous for its mouth-watering delicacies, became a hotspot for frank, supportive conversations about menopause.

Amber's journey with menopause was far from over, but she was no longer wandering in the dark. She had lit a torch, illuminating her own path and, in turn, helping others navigate their way.

In sharing Amber's journey, we glimpse the profound personal transformation that can accompany menopause. Amber's story is one of resilience and strength, of curiosity and openness. It shows us how science, personal experiences, and societal attitudes intersect, painting a multi-faceted picture of menopause. It brings us face-to-face with the knowns and unknowns of menopause, reminding us that while every woman's journey is unique, none of us are alone.

KEY TAKEAWAYS

1. Menopause, typically occurring between 45 and 55 years of age, involves significant hormonal changes.

2. Despite extensive research, areas of menopause, including its purpose and the individual responses to hormonal shifts, remain mysterious.

3. Personal reflection on societal attitudes and individual understanding of menopause is integral to one's journey.

4. Sharing real-life narratives, like Lisa's, underscores that menopause can usher in growth and positive changes.

5. Mapping personal experiences through a journal helps to better understand and navigate the unique menopausal journey.

FINAL THOUGHTS

Menopause is not an ending; it's a new chapter. It's a journey filled with its own share of trials but also opportunities for self-discovery and growth. And remember, no two journeys are the same. Just like Amber, each woman's voyage through menopause is uniquely her own.

This journey demands patience and understanding from ourselves and from those around us. It calls for embracing change, adapting, learning, and continuously growing. And yes, it also involves navigating some hot flashes and a few unexpected turns. But, as you've seen, there's much more to menopause than just the symptoms. It's a transition, a transformation, a new phase of life.

So, instead of fearing this change, let's try to understand it, accept it, and learn from it. Let's shape our menopause journey with our unique experiences and perspectives and not let it define us. Because remember, you are not just a woman going through menopause. You are a person, an individual with strengths and abilities, dreams and hopes, going through a phase of life.

As we continue our voyage in the next chapter, we'll delve into the symptoms of menopause. We'll break them down, understand them better, and explore ways to navigate through them.

THE MUDDLED MAZE OF MENOPAUSE: SYMPTOMS UNCOVERED

In our earlier rendezvous, we've untangled the facts and myths about menopause, but now it's time to confront the proverbial elephant in the room – the notorious 'symptoms'. Imagine walking into an arena where different artists are performing their solos – each unique, each impactful. That's the menopause concert in your body.

This roundabout of symptoms can often be overwhelming, and understandably so.

Symptoms of menopause, in all their diversity, can sometimes make us feel like our bodies have been hijacked. We might not recognize ourselves. But remember, just like an elaborate firework show, the chaotic beauty eventually settles into calm. And as we explore these symptoms, we aim to provide you with a flashlight in this labyrinth, a map to navigate the tide.

And remember, while these symptoms are predominantly physical, they're closely linked to our mental health. You know the feeling when you can't find your glasses only to realize they're on your head? That's brain fog. You might laugh at it now, but at the moment, it's far from amusing. It's these seemingly small things that can be a source of stress and anxiety. But hold tight as we dive deeper into the ocean of knowledge and make sense of it all.

THE HEAT WAVE: HOT FLASHES

If Menopause were a rock band, hot flashes would undoubtedly be its lead singer – standing center stage, guitar in hand, stealing the show. Imagine you're enjoying a regular day, perhaps debating the existential question of whether to indulge in a croissant or a muffin, when suddenly you're hit by an internal heatwave. A fleeting tropical vacation without the pleasure of the beach or the cocktail in your hand.

In simple terms, a hot flash is a sudden feeling of heat sweeping your body, almost like the feeling of your blood boiling minus the horror movie. You might also notice a red, flushed face and sweating, especially around your upper body. It's like your body decides to spontaneously throw a sauna party, and it forgot to give you the invite. With an unexpected start and no particular duration, hot flashes can range from being a minor annoyance to a major disruption.

The Science Behind Hot Flashes

Now, let's dive into the 'why' behind these impromptu heat sessions.

The true culprit is your changing estrogen levels, but why blame a single hormone when you can blame your entire hypothalamus? That's right, your hypothalamus - your brain's built-in thermostat - becomes a tad overzealous with these hormonal fluctuations.

As your estrogen levels ebb and flow during menopause, the hypothalamus gets mixed signals and falsely detects that your body temperature is too high. This sets off an alarm for a whole-body cool-down, causing the blood vessels near your skin to expand, a process known as vasodilation. This vasodilation is the primary driver behind the warmth and visible redness that appear during a hot flash.

Alongside this, your sweat glands are put into overdrive, hoping to cool you down through evaporation. Unfortunately, your heart also gets dragged into this mess, causing a rapid heartbeat or heart palpitations.

Research on Hot Flashes

Around 75% of menopausal women experience hot flashes, which means that in any gathering of women over 40, you're probably in the majority if you feel like you're randomly combusting from within.

Moreover, these hot flashes aren't just restricted to the menopause phase. They often stage their debut during perimenopause, the transitional period before menopause begins.

The end of hot flashes? Well, they don't abide by a strict timeline, and some women might continue to experience them for several years post-menopause.

Interestingly, researchers have found that hot flashes aren't a global phenomenon, with their prevalence significantly varying across different cultures and ethnicities. Lower rates of hot flashes have been observed in countries like Japan and Singapore as compared to the West. This variation is speculated to be due to differences in diet, lifestyle, and cultural attitudes toward menopause and aging.

And, to add another twist to the tale, did you know that all hot flashes are not 'hot' or visible? Some of you might be experiencing 'silent' hot flashes. A study using skin conductance monitors has shown that some women have hot flashes without even realizing it.

Wrapping up the hot flash saga, it's clear that these unexpected heat waves are a prominent feature of the menopausal landscape. As we navigate through this journey, it's important to remember that each woman's experience is unique. Some may need fans and cold drinks on standby, while others might just need a light cardigan.

The main goal is to keep cool — literally and figuratively.

THE RED ALARM: ABNORMAL BLEEDING

Just when you thought you'd bid adieu to the monthly red alert, menopause throws a curveball. You're triumphantly cartwheeling towards the finish line of your menstruating years, only to be tripped up by an unexpected guest—abnormal bleeding.

Now, you might be asking, "What constitutes 'abnormal' when we're talking about bleeding during menopause?" Fair question. While menopause ultimately leads to the end of your periods, the journey there can often involve a bit of a roller coaster ride when it comes to your monthly cycle. You might find yourself dealing with periods that are heavier, longer, or more frequent than usual. And in the club of menopause symptoms, this is known as abnormal uterine bleeding.

Yes, even in the face of menopause, your uterus insists on having the last word.

The Role of Uterine Fibroids

In this irregular terrain, uterine fibroids often play a villainous role. These benign growths in your uterus can sometimes be the pesky culprits behind the change in your bleeding patterns. Imagine a crowd of uninvited guests showing up at your party and causing chaos—that's fibroids for you.

Uterine fibroids can vary in size, from tiny entities that your doctor would need a microscope to see to bulky masses that can distort the shape of your uterus. These party crashers can lead to longer, more frequent, and heavier periods. Depending on your symptoms, your doctor may want to test the fibroids to ensure they aren't cancerous and potentially remove them if they are disruptive.

But before you go giving the stink eye to any potential fibroid formations, remember that they're not always the troublemakers. Other changes related to menopause can also cause irregular bleeding.

Statistics on Abnormal Bleeding

Here's a bit of trivia for you: did you know that up to 30% of women might be sharing this abnormal bleeding experience with you? Yep, it's another common entry in the menopause symptom directory.

Research has thrown up some interesting findings about abnormal uterine bleeding during menopause. Firstly, this isn't a universal experience, and secondly, the causes can vary widely. Fibroids certainly play their part in some cases, but hormonal fluctuations, polyps, endometrial atrophy (thinning of the uterine lining), or, more rarely, endometrial cancer can also cause abnormal bleeding.

Studies show that while many women experience irregular bleeding in their 40s and 50s, only a small percentage of these cases end up being due to more serious underlying conditions. So while it's important to get any changes checked out by a doctor, it's also important not to panic.

Abnormal bleeding during menopause is like that final pop quiz before summer break - you thought you were done with the hard stuff, but here comes one last challenge. It's not the most pleasant of surprises, but with a solid understanding (and perhaps a well-stocked supply of sanitary products), it's just another part of the journey to navigate.

FOGGY JUNCTION: BRAIN FOG

Let's now navigate through the mists of the mind, aka 'brain fog.' Don't you just hate it when you walk into a room and can't remember why you're there? Or when you're mid-conversation and suddenly that important thing you wanted to say has fluttered away from your brain like a rogue butterfly?

That's brain fog, ladies, a frequent gate-crasher during menopause. It's like your brain decided to take an unannounced sabbatical just when you needed it the most. The daily crossword puzzle that you used to conquer with aplomb now feels like deciphering hieroglyphics.

You'd forget your head if it wasn't screwed on tight!

How Menopause Influences the Brain

Brain fog during menopause isn't your mind playing cruel tricks on you. It's a legitimate symptom. Menopause can sometimes feel like a remote controller for your body, pushing all sorts of buttons, and the brain is no exception.

Our brains and estrogen have a deep and enduring love affair. Estrogen helps in regulating mood, controlling body temperature, and, very importantly, facilitating communication between brain cells. When menopause comes a-knocking, and estrogen levels go off-roading, the brain feels the impact.

The outcome? A foggy mind struggling with memory and concentration. It's not that the information isn't there; it just takes a bit longer to access it.

Research on Brain Fog

Research verifies this 'brain fog' phenomenon that many women experience during menopause. According to several studies, menopausal women show a tendency towards mild memory impairments, although here's the good news, it doesn't progress into a permanent state or lead to diseases like dementia.

Brain fog is one of those symptoms that's unique for everyone. Some women might experience it as forgetting common words or names, others as struggling to maintain focus. Some may only notice it for a few months, while others could have it loitering around for years.

So, what's the takeaway from all this?

Well, firstly, if you've been feeling a bit foggy, you're not alone. Secondly, this isn't a permanent foggy state. Picture it as driving through a patch of heavy fog, but eventually, you'll come out the other side into clear skies.

So the next time you find your keys in the fridge or can't remember the name of that actor—you know, the one from that movie with the thing—blame it on menopause. But remember, this fog too shall pass, and in the meantime, feel free to make the most of the phrase, "Oops, my menopause moment!"

INSOMNIAC NIGHTS: SLEEP ISSUES

Has your precious shut-eye time morphed into tossing-and-turning theater?

Welcome to another joy of menopause – sleep issues. Think of it as your body throwing a wild party every night, but you're the only one not having fun.

So why does menopause treat sleep like an unwanted guest? Once again, our beloved hormone, estrogen, is at the center of this plot. Estrogen helps us get that sweet, deep sleep. So when levels drop during menopause, our sleep quality can take a nosedive. Combine this with late-night hot flash festivals, and it's no surprise that you're clocking more hours with Netflix than in dreamland.

Common Sleep Problems

A variety of sleep problems can arise during menopause, and it's not just about struggling to fall asleep. It's also about staying asleep. For many women, nights become a series of waking up, falling back asleep, and then waking up again – a loop more tiring than any workout session.

There's also the infamous sleep apnea. This condition, characterized by pauses in breathing during sleep, can become a frequent visitor during menopause. Plus, let's not forget insomnia - the classic 'I desperately want to sleep but just can't' scenario.

Recent Findings on Sleep Issues

According to research, you're not alone in this nocturnal battle. Approximately 40%-50% of menopausal women experience some form of sleep disturbance. A study from the National Sleep Foundation found that 61% of post-menopausal women reported insomnia symptoms.

Another research tidbit – your personal furnace, aka hot flashes, can be a sleep thief. They don't always wake you up, but they can push you from deep to light sleep, making you feel exhausted the next day.

Before you resign yourself to a life of permanent under-eye bags and caffeine infusions, remember this - while menopause can be a sleep disrupter, it doesn't mean you're doomed to eternal sleepless nights. There are strategies to combat these issues, from lifestyle changes to medical treatments. So put on your battle armor, ladies – it's time to reclaim our peaceful nights from the clutches of menopause!

As we move forward, let's remember – we're not just learning about these symptoms; we're also building a roadmap to navigate through them. So next time you find yourself sheep-counting at 3 am, remember - you're not alone, and this, too, shall pass; oh, and make sure you log it in your menopause journal!

Meanwhile, enjoy the sunrise; it's a new dawn, it's a new day!

DARK CLOUDS: DEPRESSION

Alright, ladies, it's time to talk about a less visible but impactful aspect of menopause - our mental health, specifically depression. Menopause doesn't always play fair, does it? As if hot flashes and sleep disturbances weren't enough, it has to throw in a generous helping of mood swings and depression. It's like getting socks for Christmas when you were hoping for a diamond necklace.

Now, this doesn't mean that every woman who enters menopause will start humming blues tunes, but the risk of experiencing depression does increase. This can happen even if you've never had a depressive episode before. Estrogen, our hormone du jour, plays a role in regulating mood. So when these levels start see-sawing during menopause, our emotions can follow suit. Add sleep deprivation, hot flashes, weight gain, and the general stress of this major life transition, and it can create the perfect storm for depression.

Significant Studies on Depression and Menopause

Turning to our trusty scientists and their research, studies corroborate that menopause is a high-risk period for depression. One study found that women are 2-4 times more likely to experience symptoms of depression during perimenopause than before it.

Research shows that depression during menopause isn't just more common; it's also less responsive to traditional depression treatments. And it seems women with past depression episodes may have a more challenging time during menopause. This might seem like a raw deal, but remember, knowledge is power. By understanding this risk, we can prepare for it and seek help when needed.

Managing Depression During Menopause

Now, this isn't about painting a picture of doom and gloom. It's about awareness and action. There are plenty of strategies to manage depression during menopause. Here are some:

1. *Therapy*: Cognitive-behavioral therapy, a form of talk therapy, has proven to be effective. So, if you find

your mood in constant flux, remember that
therapists are friends.

2. *Antidepressants*: These may be recommended in
some cases and can also help with other menopause
symptoms.

3. *Lifestyle changes*: Regular exercise, a healthy diet,
adequate sleep, and mindfulness practices can help
regulate mood and decrease depression symptoms.

4. *Hormone Therapy*: In some cases, balancing the
hormones might help manage mood swings and
depression.

Depression is a dark cloud, no doubt. But remember, every
cloud has a silver lining. If we accept its existence and reach
out for support, we can find the sunlight again. So, let's
remember to take care of our mental health as we navigate this
menopausal journey.

We've got this, ladies!

THE SCALES TIPPING: WEIGHT GAIN

It's time to talk about the elephant in the room. Or rather,
the extra pounds on the scale that feel like an elephant. Yes,
we're talking about menopause and weight gain. It seems
like a cruel joke, doesn't it? Just as we're dealing with hot
flashes and mood swings, our favorite jeans start feeling a
bit...snug.

So, what gives?

Why does menopause seem to come with its very own expan-
sion pack? Well, let's blame it on the hormones – again. Estrogen, our old friend, plays a role in regulating body weight. As
estrogen levels dip during menopause, our bodies may

respond by storing more fat. There's also the matter of aging. As we get older, our metabolism slows down, making it easier to gain weight.

The weight gained during menopause isn't just regular weight; it's "special." And by special, I mean annoying. You see, this extra weight tends to park itself around our middle. This is known as visceral fat, and it carries a higher risk of heart disease and type 2 diabetes. The body carries two types of fat, subcutaneous fat and visceral fat. Subcutaneous fat is stored just beneath your skin, it's the kind that you can pinch between your fingers. Visceral fat is different. Visceral fat is behind your abdominal muscles and can't be seen, another gift of menopause.

Relevant Research and Findings

Now, before you start boxing up your skinny jeans and bidding them a tearful farewell, let's see what science has to say.

A study from the International Menopause Society found that hormonal changes during menopause could lead to increased abdominal fat. Another study in the Journal of Clinical Endocrinology & Metabolism found that menopausal changes lead to a redistribution of body fat, explaining our new "apple" shapes.

But here's a plot twist. Research also shows that menopause itself doesn't necessarily cause weight gain. It's the natural aging process and lifestyle changes. The hormonal changes of menopause might make you more likely to gain weight around your abdomen than around your hips and thighs. But, weight gain during menopause is not inevitable.

Studies suggest that diet and exercise can go a long way in managing this menopausal weight gain. That doesn't mean you need to sign up for a marathon or go on a celery juice diet. Simple changes like regular brisk walks and a balanced diet can make a significant difference. Try different things, and see what works. Just know that maybe what worked when you were 25 to lose weight may not work now at 45.

So, there's hope yet for our skinny jeans!

LEAKY PIPES: BLADDER ISSUES

If you've been finding yourself having an internal battle with your bladder, wondering if you should install a GPS for the nearest restroom, then welcome to the leaky pipes section! Menopause can have you reminiscing about the good old days when you could sneeze, laugh, or exercise without a 'urine comes out surprise.' But fear not! Understanding the why and the how can be the first step to regaining control.

Urinary issues during menopause can manifest as frequency (rushing to the bathroom every half hour), urgency (feeling like you need to go NOW), and incontinence (when the 'now' happens before you can make it to the restroom).

But why is your bladder acting like a rebellious teenager refusing to obey the rules?

Well, once again, we can point our finger at the usual suspect: estrogen. This hormone has a vital role in maintaining the health of the bladder and urethra. When estrogen levels drop during menopause, these tissues lose elasticity, leading to those unwelcome changes in urinary function. Your bladder, once a resilient water balloon, now seems to have the capacity of a shot glass.

Research on Menopause and Urinary Symptoms

According to several studies, you are definitely not alone in this.

A study in the American Journal of Obstetrics and Gynecology found that 70% of women reported an increase in urinary frequency during menopause, while 54% reported urgency and 37% experienced incontinence. Another study in the Journal of Women's Health concluded that "menopausal transition is strongly associated with prevalent and incident urinary incontinence." So, yes, it's a thing, and no, it's not just you.

Now, before you start investing in companies manufacturing bladder control products, let's explore the solutions. Many researchers are looking at ways to help menopausal women have fewer "I gotta go" moments. These range from pelvic floor exercises (Kegels, anyone?) to medication, hormone therapy, and even surgical options.

The good news is urinary issues are treatable. By talking to your healthcare provider, you can explore options that work best for you. So, next time your bladder tries to send you running, you can put up a 'not so fast' sign.

THUNDERSTORM AHEAD: MIGRAINES

Ever felt like a tiny gremlin is hammering away inside your skull, turning your brain into a pounding disco of pain? Ah, the joy of migraines! If you're already a member of the Migraine Club, menopause might just decide to amp up the VIP treatment for you.

A migraine is not just a severe headache; it's a full-fledged neurological event, complete with light sensitivity, nausea, and even visual disturbances – a true sensory circus if you will. And when menopause comes a-knocking, those hormonal fluctuations can be like an all-access pass for migraines to party harder.

Estrogen, our hormone of the hour, is again a key player here. It has a considerable influence on our brain chemicals that manage pain. As estrogen levels roller-coaster during peri-menopause, it can trigger migraines or, for the already initi-ated, increase the frequency and intensity. So, it's less of a gentle carousel ride and more of a hardcore rollercoaster one.

Research Findings on Menopause and Migraines

Let's crunch some numbers here.

According to the Migraine Research Foundation, migraines affect a whopping 39 million people in the U.S., and guess what? Women are three times more likely to experience them than men. Oh, the perks of womanhood!

And if you're thinking, "I've never had a migraine, I'll be just fine," menopause might still have a surprise for you. Studies show that migraines can make their grand debut during peri-menopause. In fact, the American Migraine Foundation suggests that women with a history of hormonal headaches can experience a significant increase during the transition to menopause.

The link between estrogen and migraines is so well established that some scientists even consider migraines a symptom of perimenopause. Fun times, right? But don't stock up on ice packs just yet; there's a silver lining here too. For many women, migraines improve after they've crossed into post-menopause territory.

Just hang in there; the thunderstorm does pass!

BEDROOM BLUES: SEX ISSUES

Imagine this: one minute, you're frolicking in a lush tropical forest, and the next, you're stranded in the Mojave desert. Yep, that pretty much sums up the impact menopause can have on your sex life. But before you panic-buy a lifetime supply of lubricant and pray to the love gods, let's take a deep dive into the science of sexual changes during menopause.

Menopause, bless her heart, likes to juggle your hormones like circus balls, and your sex life, unfortunately, can become a part of this circus. The showstopper here is estrogen. As this star performer starts taking its final bows, things on stage (i.e., your body) might go a bit awry.

Estrogen, you see, is the prima donna that keeps your vaginal tissues healthy and elastic and your natural lubrication on point. But with menopause dropping the curtain on estrogen, you're left with vaginal dryness and discomfort during sex. Couple the vaginal dryness and discomfort with other symptoms such as hot flashes, mood swings, and sleep disturbances. Together, these can lead to a significantly lowered sex drive.

But worry not! This isn't the end of your sexcapades, but merely an intermission. Like any good show, things can still pick up in the second act!

Research on Sex and Menopause

Now, it's time for a quick trivia break.

The Study of Women's Health Across the Nation (SWAN) found that nearly half of the women experienced a dip in sexual desire post-menopause, while about a quarter of them had lubrication issues. But remember ladies, these are just statistics. Menopause, like a modern artist, likes to express herself differently in each woman.

But here comes the plot twist.

While menopause can meddle with your sexual health, it doesn't have to write the script for your sex life. Plenty of women have encore performances (pun totally intended) post-menopause. Being freed from the menstrual cycle drama and the pregnancy scare subplot can actually make sex more enjoyable. Yes, you heard it right, menopause can be the unexpected hero of your sexual narrative!

The sex-menopause saga doesn't end here. Research even suggests that staying sexually active can help keep some of the sexual symptoms of menopause at bay. Yes, that's right! More sex equals less discomfort. Kind of like how more chocolate equals less sadness, isn't it?

So, what's the takeaway here? Menopause may be a tricky director to work with, but you're the star of your own sexual health. Explore, adapt, and remember, every good performance involves a bit of improvisation!

THINNING THREADS: HAIR LOSS

Crowning glory losing its sheen? Hairbrush starting to look like a porcupine? It seems like menopause has brought along a rather hairy problem—hair loss.

The drama of menopause is quite like a Shakespearean play, and in this act, we have the leading lady, Estrogen, bidding us adieu. Estrogen, the fairy godmother of hair, keeps our locks lush and lustrous. When she takes a bow and exits the stage during menopause, your hair might just follow suit.

Losing some hair daily is normal, but during menopause, your shower drain might start looking like a furball. And it's not just on your head. You might notice fewer strokes with your razor as leg hair thins out too. But hey, look on the bright side: fewer shaving nicks!

Studies on Menopause and Hair Thinning

Now, let's sprinkle in some science here.

Research indicates that up to 40% of women experience hair thinning after menopause. There's a buzzword for it, too: female pattern hair loss or FPHL, if you're into the whole brevity thing.

A study in the British Journal of Dermatology showed that menopausal women with FPHL have lower estrogen and progesterone levels. Also, while you might blame your genes for your receding hairline, hormones play a crucial role too. Studies suggest that a certain pesky enzyme that converts testosterone to a hair-unfriendly hormone ramps up during menopause. So, it's not just about losing estrogen; it's also about the hormonal changing of the guard.

This thinning plot might seem a bit grim, but remember, it's not your final act. There are a plethora of treatments, therapies, and even some stylish hats that can help you steal the show. Because no matter what menopause throws your way, you're still the star of your life's play.

So, what's the takeaway from this hairy tale? Menopause is full of twists and turns, but with a bit of humor, a lot of science, and an endless supply of scrunchies, you'll get through it. Hair today, gone tomorrow, but hey, there's always wigs!

Now, onto the next curious case of menopausal phenomena. Are you ready to comb through the facts? Because we're just getting to the root of it!

CREAKY JOINTS: ACHES AND PAINS

Wake up, yawn, stretch, and...Ouch! If you're groaning more than a disgruntled teenager during these morning rituals, welcome to the "Creaky Joints Club," one of the less-advertised perks of menopause.

Did you ever imagine there'd be a day when 'feeling your age' wouldn't just be about not understanding TikTok trends but also literally feeling it in your bones? If menopause had a slogan, it might be "Experience the magic of aging...overnight!"

So, let's pop into our 'physical complaints' hat and pull out a joint issue. This is not your garden-variety "I've carried too many grocery bags" ache. No, we're talking about pain that persists longer than your spouse's snoring. This discomfort could span your back, your hips, your knees, and even your hands. In short, you could feel like a life-sized game of Operation!

Now, don't go pointing fingers at arthritis just yet. These aches and pains are also, quite conveniently, menopause's accomplices. Estrogen, that miracle worker, also helped keep inflammation in check. With it stepping back, your body may feel like a rusty Tin Man, needing a good oiling.

Research on Menopause and Joint Pain

Now, let's have a look-see at what the scientists in the white coats have to say. Studies suggest that up to 60% of post-menopausal women report joint pain. Now that's a statistic you'd rather not be a part of, right?

A study published in Climacteric, The Journal of the International Menopause Society (yes, there is such a thing, and no, it's not just Sudoku and crossword puzzles) found that menopausal women were more likely to have hand pain and poorer hand function.

The Journal of Aging and Health reported an association between menopause and chronic knee pain. So, it seems, menopause could give you a 'knee-slapper' of a time, but without the fun joke part.

Meanwhile, a North American Menopause Society (NAMS) survey of 2,000 women found that women with menopause symptoms are nearly twice as likely to have chronic pain. Talk about adding insult to injury!

But, before you feel like an old rickety bridge, remember, there's a lot you can do to keep your joints jumping. A bit of exercise, some healthy eating, and a lot of can-do attitude can make a world of difference. So, next time you feel a creak or a groan, just tell your joints: "Ain't nobody got time for that!"

Menopause is an adventure, my friend. There are surprises around every corner, and while some of them might make you groan a little, remember: you're not alone in this. The "Creaky Joints Club" is quite a big one, and we're all here to support each other!

KEY TAKEAWAYS

1. Menopause, while a universal stage in a woman's life, is a unique experience for everyone, with symptoms varying widely in type, intensity, and duration.
2. Hot flashes, abnormal bleeding, brain fog, sleep issues, depression, weight gain, bladder problems, sexual issues, migraines, hair loss, and aches are some common symptoms that women may experience during menopause.

3. Menopause is a result of hormonal shifts in the body, especially a decrease in estrogen levels, which can affect everything from your mood to your metabolism.

4. Research suggests all these symptoms are common signs of menopause.

5. While many symptoms can cause discomfort or distress, remember they are part of a natural process, and numerous strategies and treatments are available to help manage them.

FINAL THOUGHTS

In the theatre of life, menopause might seem like an act you'd rather skip. Yet, here it is – an unavoidable encore to the fertile years. But remember, this isn't a tragedy; it's a rite of passage that every woman shares. You're not alone on this stage.

Change can be unsettling, even scary, but it can also be a catalyst for growth and renewal. So, take a deep breath, step into the spotlight, and embrace this new act with courage and resilience. No symptom is too big or small to seek help for, and there's no shame in voicing your experiences or reaching out to medical professionals. This is your body, your performance, and you have the power to navigate this transition in a way that makes you feel most comfortable.

Menopause is indeed a change, but it isn't a curtain call on your well-being or zest for life. Like any scene change, it offers a chance to reassess, adapt, and improvise. You might just find that the best is yet to come!

From hot flashes to brain fog, from weight gain to mood swings, we've talked about the various ways menopause can impact your body and mind. But menopause isn't a one-way street. In our next chapter, "Taking the Reins: Managing Menopausal Symptoms," we'll discuss actionable strategies and treatments to help you navigate this transition with confidence and ease. So, buckle up and get ready to take control of your menopause journey!

NOW WHAT? AN ACTION PLAN FOR MENOPAUSE SYMPTOMS

Welcome to the "Now What?" chapter of this wild menopause ride. Or, as I like to call it, "So you're menopausal, now let's get down to business." You're not just surviving the menopause jungle; you're gearing up to conquer it.

You see, when life gives you menopause, you can sit around feeling hot and bothered (and not in the fun way), or you can grab life by the lapels and say, "Alright, menopause, show me what you've got!" This chapter is all about that latter approach.

Now that we've dissected the what, why, and how of menopause (without the use of any actual scalpels, thankfully), let's delve into the "now what?" This is where we roll up our sleeves and dive into a buffet of strategies that can help you manage your menopause symptoms.

The exciting bit is that there isn't a one-size-fits-all approach. Just as you've got your own unique fashion sense (that may or may not involve bedazzled sweatpants), your menopause management strategy will be just as unique to you. From hormone therapy to lifestyle changes, alternative therapies, medications, and complementary therapies, we've got a smorgasbord of options that's as diverse as an all-you-can-eat buffet at a Las Vegas casino.

So, whether you're a risk-taker looking to hit the jackpot with hormone therapy or you prefer to play it safe with lifestyle changes, we've got you covered. Heck, you could even dabble in alternative therapies if you're feeling adventurous. No judgment here.

Just remember, navigating through menopause is a journey, and it's one you don't have to take alone. Just consider this chapter as your friendly tour guide, offering you the top attractions, hidden gems, and even some potential tourist traps. Get ready to chart your path and embark on your adventure.

Because, in the end, menopause isn't a monster. It's just an uninvited guest that's overstayed its welcome, and with the right approach, you might just find it isn't so bad. So grab a cup of chamomile tea (or a glass of wine, I'm not policing your beverage choices), and let's explore this together.

Your "Now What" journey begins...well, now!

LIFESTYLE CHANGES: THE POWER IN YOUR HANDS

Alright, ladies, grab your capes. It's time for some superhero-level lifestyle adaptations. Why, you ask? Because lifestyle changes are the secret weapon that helps manage menopause symptoms. No, they can't perform miracles, but they sure can ease the ride. From your diet to your Zumba class, to that chill yoga session, and even the Friday glass of red wine – they all play a part in this grand symphony we call menopause.

So, let's conduct this orchestra, shall we? Let's take charge, tweak a few habits, maybe introduce some new ones, and show menopause who's boss!

The Impact of Lifestyle Changes on Menopause

Understanding the impact of lifestyle changes on menopause is akin to unlocking a door to personal empowerment during this phase of life. Knowing what habits can exacerbate or alleviate menopausal symptoms gives women an actionable toolkit to navigate their menopausal journey better.

When we grasp the pivotal role that lifestyle plays in our overall health, particularly during periods of significant hormonal shifts like menopause, we can develop strategies to optimize our well-being. It provides a proactive approach to health, allowing us to anticipate potential issues and counter them with lifestyle adjustments. This is not just about reducing the intensity of hot flashes or improving sleep quality but also about enhancing our overall quality of life.

The significance of understanding lifestyle changes also lies in the opportunity it presents for preventative health. For instance, weight management and regular exercise have well-established benefits for cardiovascular health, a concern that becomes more prominent post-menopause due to the protective effect of estrogen dwindling.

Additionally, being cognizant of the lifestyle-menopause link helps in creating a holistic approach to health. It discourages over-reliance on medical interventions and encourages a balance between physical, emotional, and mental health. This could mean adopting mindfulness practices for stress relief, improving dietary habits, or incorporating regular physical activity.

In essence, understanding the influence of lifestyle changes offers an essential compass to guide you through the journey of menopause. It allows for the proactive management of symptoms and underpins a broader, holistic approach to health during this phase of life.

Suggested Lifestyle Changes

Well, it's time to dive into the nitty-gritty, the fun part, the big kahuna of managing menopause. How, you ask?

With a few tweaks here and a couple of additions there. It's like conducting a lifestyle symphony – a little more violin here (in the form of veggies), a little less trumpet there (bye-bye cigarettes!). Let's chart out some lifestyle changes that could make your menopause journey less of a rickety roller coaster ride and more of a scenic Ferris wheel.

Your Plate is Your Palette: Eating Healthy

First things first, let's address your plate. Think of it as your canvas and your foods as the colors you can use to paint your health picture. How vibrant and healthy do you want it to be?

Incorporating plenty of fruits, vegetables, lean proteins, and whole grains can be the artistic stroke you need. Try adding foods that contain plant estrogens, such as broccoli, cauliflower, dark berries, chickpeas, and soybeans. These nutrients act like the engine oil that keeps your body machinery humming smoothly. Remember the notorious villain in our menopause saga? Yep, I'm talking about the declining estrogen levels. To combat the bone loss associated with reduced estrogen levels, calcium, magnesium, and vitamin D need to make frequent appearances in your diet. It's like inviting Batman and Superman to your party. Can it get any cooler?

But beware of processed foods! They're like wolves in sheep's clothing, luring you with their convenience and speed but wreaking havoc on your health. Our advice? Embrace the periphery of your grocery store, where the fresh produce lives, and treat the inner aisles like a lava-filled obstacle course.

Move Those Muscles: The Exercise Factor

It's time to get moving. If exercise were a pill, it would be the kind of wonder drug that pharmaceutical companies would fight tooth and nail over. The benefits? Almost too many to count. It can help maintain a healthy weight, keep your heart ticking like a Swiss watch, improve sleep (who doesn't love a good night's rest?), and even boost your mood.

You don't need to train like you're competing for an Olympic medal. Aim for at least 150 minutes of moderate exercise per week. This can be as simple as a brisk walk with your dog, a dance-off with your grandkids, or a bike ride through your local park. The key is consistency and enjoyment - pick something you love, and the exercise will be the cherry on top.

There are a variety of programs out there that target menopause weight gain. I pretty much have tried them all. My three key takeaways are 1. what worked when you were 25 no longer works at 45, 2. try different things, and 3. killing yourself with cardio will only make you miserable and cause you to gain weight. Menopausal diet and weight loss is an entire topic that can fill its own book, so that's what I'm doing; stay tuned for the next book in the series... "*Menopause Makeover: The Ultimate Diet and Exercise Guide for a Vibrant You!*" coming soon.

Mind over Mood: Stress Management

Next on our hit list is stress. Life throws us curveballs – daily deadlines, traffic jams, argumentative teens - and menopause might feel like another tricky pitch. But remember, stress doesn't get to call the shots; you do. Stress management techniques like yoga, deep breathing, or even a relaxing painting session can be your shield in the face of stress-induced triggers.

Try out different techniques and find what works for you. It's your personal stress-busting recipe – add a pinch of meditation, a dollop of deep breathing, and maybe even a sprinkle of tai chi. And voila! You have your custom-made stress management plan.

The Drama Duo: Limiting Alcohol and Avoiding Smoking

The last change on our list addresses two key culprits in the menopause saga: alcohol and tobacco. While that glass of wine might seem like the perfect unwind after a long day, and cigarettes might have been a longtime companion, they don't mix well with menopause. In fact, they could amplify symptoms and create new problems.

Limit your alcohol intake (I know this is easier said than done), and if you smoke, now would be a great time to call it quits. There are numerous resources available to help, from apps and hotlines to support groups.

So there you have it, ladies. Your menopause lifestyle transformation plan. Remember, it's not about perfection but progress. Maybe you can't ditch your chocolate habit entirely, but you can substitute dark chocolate instead of milk chocolate. Perhaps you can't make it to the gym every day, but you can take a longer walk during lunch breaks.

So, let's make menopause the start of an incredible new chapter – the chapter where you take control and develop the habit of consistency. Now, who's ready to rock this menopause party?

ALTERNATIVE THERAPIES: THE ROAD LESS TRAVELED

Have you ever found yourself at a crossroads, with the familiar path beckoning on one side and the less traveled, mysterious one tempting you from the other?

Menopause can feel like that, with traditional paths of treatment on the one hand and a whole new world of alternative therapies on the other. Let's stroll down this less-traveled path together and explore what it has to offer. No breadcrumbs are required, I promise!

Understanding Alternative Therapies

Alternative therapies are like the indie band of the medical world. They may not be mainstream, but they have a loyal fanbase, and their popularity is on the rise. Also, just like indie bands, they can offer some unique and fresh tunes when you're tired of hearing the same old songs.

In essence, alternative therapies are methods of treatment that aren't part of conventional Western medical practice. They're kind of like the rebel cousin who ditched the family business to go backpacking around the world and came back with a treasure trove of unique wisdom and experiences.

Some examples of alternative therapies include acupuncture, herbal medicine, massage, biofeedback, and yoga. Now, before you start worrying that this means trekking up a remote mountain to find a hermit yogi (although, if that's your thing, more power to you!), let me clarify. Many of these treatments can be found right in your neighborhood – at local clinics, wellness centers, or even through online platforms.

Why are they used, you ask? Well, for one, they provide another set of tools in our toolbox for managing menopause symptoms. Also, they often focus on treating the whole person, not just the symptoms. It's a bit like gardening. Instead of just watering the wilting leaves, these therapies aim to nourish the roots, believing that healthy roots will naturally lead to a healthy plant.

And let's not forget the appeal of a more natural route. When you've had your fill of pharmaceutical concoctions, the idea of using herbs, movements, or energy to manage your symptoms can feel like a breath of fresh air. It's kind of like choosing between a lab-produced vitamin pill and a juicy, fresh orange – both have their place, but there's something inherently appealing about the natural option.

But don't just take my word for it. Let's dig a bit deeper and discover what science has to say about some of these alternative therapies and their effectiveness in managing menopause symptoms.

Exploring Different Alternative Therapies

Have you ever seen an acupuncture doll? It's like a voodoo doll, but instead of casting curses, it's all about healing. Covered with tiny marks indicating pressure points, it's a map of the body's superhighway of energy. But instead of being terrifyingly creepy, it's... well, okay, it's still a little creepy. But, it's also a testament to a medical practice that's been around for over 2000 years. Who's ready to roll up their sleeves and get a little prickly?

Acupuncture: No, this is not about turning you into a human pin cushion! Those tiny, thin needles stimulate specific points in your body, also known as meridians. Think of it as poking your body's energy into motion. Scientific research shows that acupuncture can be beneficial in managing hot flashes, sleep disturbances, and mood swings during menopause. It's like having your personal thermostat, sleep aid, and mood booster all rolled into one! Just remember, with acupuncture, just like with any other medical procedure, the experience of the practitioner matters. Make sure you find a well-qualified practitioner.

Next, let's dive into the leafy green world of herbs. Imagine if your spice rack were a team of superheroes, each with their own superpowers. Well, in the world of herbal medicine, that's pretty much the reality!

Herbal Remedies: These are nature's very own medicine cabinet. They're like the cool, hipster chefs who've been creating organic, locally-sourced, health-boosting recipes long before it was trendy. Common herbs used for managing menopausal symptoms include black cohosh, red clover, and St. John's Wort. They sound like characters in a fairy tale, but they're serious contenders in the fight against menopause symptoms. They've been studied for their effects on everything from hot flashes to mood swings. Remember, though, that even natural remedies can have side effects and interact with other medications, so always discuss with a healthcare provider before starting any new treatment.

And now for something completely different and somewhat controversial. Step right up and witness the amazing world of homeopathy!

Homeopathy: Homeopathy operates on the "like cures like" principle. It's the medical equivalent of fighting fire with fire, only without the potential for third-degree burns. While some folks swear by it, the scientific jury is still out, with many studies finding no effect beyond placebo. That said, for some women, it can provide relief from menopausal symptoms like hot flashes, night sweats, and mood swings. If nothing else, the tiny, sugar-coated pellets make you feel like you're in a Harry Potter potion class.

So, there you have it! A whistle-stop tour of the wide world of alternative therapies. But remember, the alternative route isn't for everyone, and that's okay. Like choosing between a guided tour and off-roading, it's about finding what fits best for you.

RESEARCH AND EVIDENCE ON ALTERNATIVE THERAPIES

Let's start by acknowledging the 800-pound gorilla in the room: alternative therapies can be a bit...well, controversial. Some folks swear by them like they swear by their grandma's apple pie recipe, while others are more skeptical, raising an eyebrow higher than Spock on Star Trek.

But here's the thing: when it comes to navigating menopause, our goal is to keep all options on the table and let science do the talking.

Acupuncture: Getting to the Point

Acupuncture is like the classic rock band of alternative therapies; it's been around forever and still manages to draw a crowd. Several studies have investigated its impact on menopausal symptoms, especially those pesky hot flashes.

In 2016, a review of multiple studies found that acupuncture reduced the frequency and severity of hot flashes for some women. However, before you rush to lie down on a bed of needles, remember that results can vary. Some women felt like they had won the symptom-relief lottery, while others noticed no significant difference.

Science, like life, is complicated.

Herbal Remedies: Sowing Seeds of Hope

When it comes to the science behind herbal remedies, the landscape is as diverse as an Amazonian rainforest. Black cohosh, a native North American plant, is one of the most studied. Black Cohosh is used in Native American herbal medicine to treat a variety of illnesses. Some research suggests it may help reduce hot flashes and mood swings, but other studies beg to differ.

Red clover, another popular plant in the herbal remedy game, has shown mixed results in scientific trials but is frequently used to treat or prevent various menopause symptoms, including hot flashes, night sweats, and bone loss.

When it comes to helping boost your sex drive, Ashwagandha root may stimulate your libido and increase your satisfaction by increasing blood flow to your lady bits. Maca Root, which is high in zinc, an essential mineral for sex hormones, may help as well.

In the end, it seems that Mother Nature likes to keep some of her secrets, well, secret.

Homeopathy: The Placebo Debate

Ah, homeopathy, the Marmite of alternative therapies—you either love it or you hate it.

Homeopathy is based on the belief that the body can cure itself. The idea is to stimulate the healing process by using tiny amounts of plants and minerals to stimulate healing.

In the scientific community, homeopathy has been controversial, mainly because many studies find its effects comparable to a placebo. You know, the sugar pill dressed up as a magic cure in clinical trials.

However, some women find that homeopathy helps manage their symptoms. Again do your research and talk to a Homeopath. After all, if you feel better, does it matter if it was the remedy or the placebo effect? It's a question as philosophical as it is scientific!

What's clear is that research into alternative therapies is like exploring a new frontier. There are exciting discoveries, unexpected dead-ends, and a whole lot of unknown territory. However, with an open mind and a critical eye, we can navigate this landscape and make informed choices about our health.

MEDICATIONS: THE MODERN MEDICINE APPROACH

Welcome to the world of modern medicine, the land of science-backed solutions, lab coats, and a pill for every ill (or so it seems). When it comes to navigating the choppy waters of menopause, it's a bit like being given a map and a compass, only the map keeps changing, and the compass... well, let's just say it's not always pointing north.

But fear not; our medicinal boat is equipped with more than just hormone therapy. So, buckle up as we dive into the marvels of modern pharmacology to explore the medicinal approach to tackling menopause. From the famous hormone therapy to the unsung heroes of non-hormonal treatments, I'm about to lift the lid on your medicine cabinet and see what's really going on inside.

Non-Hormonal Medications for Menopause

If hormone therapy were a high school, it'd be the popular jock, the homecoming queen, and the class president all rolled into one. But just as high school is more than just prom queens and touchdowns, so too is the realm of menopause medications.

Step aside, hormones; it's time to shine the spotlight on some unexpected guests that have RSVP'd to the menopausal party - non-hormonal medications. These underdogs in the pharmacological world are stepping up their game and offering women more options than ever.

Antidepressants: Not Just for Your Mood Anymore

When you think of antidepressants, hot flash relief probably isn't the first thing that comes to mind. But surprise! Selective serotonin reuptake inhibitors (SSRIs) and serotonin and norepinephrine reuptake inhibitors (SNRIs) aren't just for combating depression - they've been shown to reduce the frequency of hot flashes, too. It's like ordering a salad and finding out it comes with a free slice of cheesecake. Except the cheesecake is hot flash relief, and the salad is improved mood. This analogy might have gotten away from me...

Gabapentin: From Seizures to Sweat Relief

Originally used to treat seizures, Gabapentin is the poster child for the phrase "unexpected benefits." While it might not have been voted "Most Likely to Reduce Hot Flashes" in medical school, it's definitely proving the doubters wrong now. In several studies, Gabapentin has shown promise in reducing hot flashes, although it can cause side effects like dizziness and fatigue. And let's be honest, who needs extra dizziness in their menopause journey?

Clonidine: A Blood Pressure Medication's Second Act

Once upon a time, Clonidine was just a humble blood pressure medication. Now, it's taking a star turn on the menopause stage by reducing hot flashes. It's like finding out your unassuming accountant neighbor is actually a brilliant violinist. However, side effects can include dry mouth, constipation, and sleep disturbances. So, it's not quite the Beethoven's Symphony of Medications, but it might just help keep those hot flashes in check.

Osteoporosis Medications: Your Bones' Best Friends

With estrogen levels dropping faster than my cell phone battery, bone loss can be a real concern during menopause. Enter: osteoporosis medications. These bone warriors help maintain bone density and reduce the risk of fractures. Think of them as the personal trainers for your skeleton, helping it stay strong and healthy.

Whether they were initially designed for menopause or not, these non-hormonal medications have been invited to the party and are starting to make their mark. So, if hormone therapy isn't your cup of tea, fear not; there are plenty of other brews to try.

Remember, variety is the spice of life, even when it comes to navigating menopause. In the end, the best medication for you is the one that suits your symptoms, lifestyle, and body.

Benefits and Risks of Non-Hormonal Medications

Picture yourself in a modern art museum, standing in front of a canvas splashed with vivid colors and bold shapes. Some people might see chaos, while others might see a masterpiece. Non-hormonal medications for menopause can be viewed in much the same way. There are undeniable benefits, but there are also some risks that come with the territory. Like abstract art, the effectiveness of these treatments can be subjective and varies from person to person.

First, let's take a stroll down the sunlit side of the gallery and explore the potential benefits. Non-hormonal treatments, such as certain antidepressants, anti-seizure medications, and blood pressure drugs, have been shown to reduce the frequency and severity of hot flashes. And let's be honest, who wouldn't want to put a damper on those uninvited bursts of heat disrupting your day (or night)?

In particular, certain selective serotonin reuptake inhibitors (SSRIs) and serotonin and norepinephrine reuptake inhibitors (SNRIs), often used to treat depression, have been found effective in alleviating hot flashes. Talk about a two-for-one special, right? These antidepressants could not only help keep your internal thermostat in check but also aid in managing mood swings often associated with menopause.

Another non-hormonal superstar on the list is Gabapentin, an anti-seizure medication which has shown a knack for cooling down hot flashes. It's like having a personal air conditioner that kicks in just when you need it.

Then there's Clonidine, a medication originally used to treat high blood pressure. Now, you may be wondering, what on earth does blood pressure have to do with menopause? Well, Clonidine, in its free time, moonlights as a hot flash suppressant, reducing their frequency and intensity. It's like the Clark Kent of menopause treatments.

Now, let's dim the lights and venture into the other side of the gallery – the risks and side effects. Like every medication, non-hormonal treatments can come with potential side effects and interactions. SSRIs and SNRIs, for instance, can cause nausea, insomnia, and a dry mouth and might not play nice with other medications you're taking.

Gabapentin, while effective, can cause dizziness, fatigue, and balance problems in some women. It's like being on a merry-go-round without the merry part. And Clonidine, our high blood pressure hero, may cause dry mouth, constipation, or drowsiness.

Not to mention, these medications, like any others, can have different effects on different people, and their effectiveness can vary. It's kind of like a game of medication roulette, where you hope you're placing your bets on the right treatment.

Remember, non-hormonal medications are not a one-size-fits-all solution. The right medication for you will depend on your symptoms, overall health, and personal preference. It's crucial to have an open discussion with your healthcare provider about your options, benefits, and potential risks to make an informed decision.

In our gallery of non-hormonal medications, we have seen that these treatments, like abstract art, can be a mixture of chaos and beauty. They offer potential relief from menopausal symptoms but come with their own set of potential risks. The key is to find what works best for you - your masterpiece in the canvas of menopause treatment options. And remember, even Picasso didn't paint his masterpiece in a day. It's a process, and finding the right treatment might take some time and patience, but with the right guidance, you'll find your way.

Real-Life Applications of Medications

Imagine you're watching a movie where the main character is tasked with battling a formidable foe. Our heroine in this film is "Menopause". She's strong, she's relentless, and she's armed with an array of medications as her secret weapons. Let's grab some popcorn and watch as these medical marvels spring into action in real life.

In the first scene, we meet Carol, a corporate lawyer who's battling sleep-disrupting night sweats. For Carol, her bedroom was less a haven of rest and more like a tropical rainforest, leaving her exhausted during the day. A chance discussion with her healthcare provider introduced her to the world of SSRIs. A couple of weeks into taking Paroxetine, a low-dose SSRI, she noticed a significant reduction in her night sweats.

Instead of waking up to change her drenched PJs, she was now sleeping through the night, and her energy levels during the day soared. Carol's story underscores the power of these medications in combating some of menopause's most notorious symptoms. And she didn't even have to hire a rainforest guide!

In the next scene, we meet Susan, a teacher who started experiencing frequent, intense hot flashes after entering menopause. The hot flashes were so severe they made her feel like she was living on the sun's surface! She was introduced to Gabapentin by her healthcare provider. After a few weeks of using this anti-seizure medication, her hot flashes diminished in both frequency and intensity. Now Susan feels more like she's living on Earth rather than the sun. Thanks, Gabapentin!

In another act of our menopause movie, we find Angela, a musician who had been struggling with mood swings so intense they could put a rollercoaster to shame. Angela found her secret weapon in the form of Venlafaxine, an SNRI. It not only helped to mellow out her mood swings but also brought down the frequency of her hot flashes. With her moods now hitting fewer high and low notes, Angela could focus on creating beautiful music instead of constantly riding the hormonal wave.

Finally, we meet Linda, a bookstore owner whose menopausal symptoms were running rampant. She was dealing with hot flashes, night sweats, and an overall decrease in her quality of life. Clonidine, initially developed for treating high blood pressure, became her ally in the menopause battlefield. With Clonidine in her corner, Linda saw a decrease in the severity and frequency of her hot flashes and started enjoying life again, one book at a time.

While all of these stories may seem like happy endings, remember that these are real-life applications, not fairy tales. Medications, whether hormonal or non-hormonal, can have side effects and may not work the same way for everyone. Our heroines Carol, Susan, Angela, and Linda found what worked for them through trial, error and open communication with their healthcare providers. Their stories highlight the importance of individualized treatment in managing menopause symptoms - there is no one-size-fits-all solution.

Whether you find yourself in a scene similar to Carol, Susan, Angela, or Linda, remember that your menopause journey is uniquely yours. It might take a bit of trial and error to find the right combination of lifestyle changes, medications, or alternative therapies that work for you. But, just like in our movie, the heroine – that's you – can come out triumphant in the end.

COMPLEMENTARY THERAPIES: THE BEST OF BOTH WORLDS

Alright, class, it's time for a pop quiz! When you hear the term "complementary therapies," do you think of:

A) Therapies that say nice things to each other? "Hey, Acupuncture, you're really on point today!"

B) Therapies that go together like peanut butter and jelly?

C) Therapies that combine conventional medical treatments with alternative therapies?

D) All of the above?

If you guessed C, you're correct! (Although, if you answered D, we appreciate your sense of humor.)

Understanding Complementary Therapies

Complementary therapies refer to a group of diverse medical and healthcare systems, practices, and products that are not generally considered part of conventional medicine but are used alongside it. Picture a medical tool belt filled with a mix of traditional tools, like medications and surgeries, and then add in a few unconventional gadgets, like acupuncture needles, yoga mats, or herbal teas. These unconventional tools might not be the first thing a doctor reaches for, but they can be incredibly useful in certain situations.

"But why would someone want to use complementary therapies?" you may ask. Excellent question, dear reader! There are many reasons why someone might choose to go this route. For starters, it's all about customization. Like ordering a tailor-made suit instead of grabbing one off the rack, complementary therapies can be personalized to meet an individual's unique needs and preferences.

For many people going through menopause, the symptoms aren't just physical – they're mental and emotional as well. And while traditional medicine does a great job of addressing the physical symptoms, it often comes up short when dealing with the mental and emotional aspects. That's where complementary therapies can really shine. Whether it's using meditation to manage stress, acupuncture to reduce hot flashes, or herbal supplements to improve sleep, these therapies can provide a more holistic approach to managing menopause.

Plus, there's the element of control. Menopause can often feel like a wild rollercoaster ride that you didn't sign up for. Complementary therapies can offer a sense of control in this often chaotic period. It's like being given the reins to steer the rollercoaster instead of just hanging on for dear life.

So, now that we know what complementary therapies are and why they're used let's roll up our sleeves and dive a bit deeper into what these therapies can offer. Get ready because we're about to dive into an ocean filled with everything from acupuncture needles to yoga mats, herbal supplements to mindfulness techniques. It's going to be an exciting journey, so buckle up and let's get started!

Different Types of Complementary Therapies

Prepare to embark on a whirlwind tour of the world of complementary therapies. Strap yourself in and keep your arms and legs inside the vehicle at all times because we're about to hit some unexpected twists and turns!

Yoga: Let's start with yoga, a practice that might be older than your great-great-great grandmother's secret cookie recipe. Originating from ancient India, yoga combines physical postures, breathing exercises, and meditation to promote physical and mental well-being. It's like a three-for-one deal on managing menopause symptoms. Regular yoga practice can help manage weight, reduce stress, and even alleviate hot flashes. All you need is a mat, some comfy clothes, and a willingness to twist your body into positions you never thought possible.

Massage: Ah, massage. Even the word sounds relaxing. Who wouldn't want to lay on a comfortable table while a professional works out the kinks in your shoulders? But it's not just about pampering yourself (though that's a pretty nice perk). Research suggests massage can help reduce symptoms like anxiety and depression and even improve sleep. Just imagine walking out of a massage session feeling like a wet noodle in a zen garden. Now, that's what I call relaxation!

Meditation: Next up, meditation. No, it's not just for bald guys in orange robes. It's a practice anyone can use to help calm the mind and body. Imagine you're a surfer, and your thoughts are the waves. Sometimes they're massive and choppy; other times, they're small and gentle. Meditation teaches you how to ride these waves instead of getting knocked over by them. It's an effective tool for managing the stress and anxiety that can come with menopause. Plus, you can do it anywhere, anytime. Stuck in traffic? Meditate. Waiting in line at the grocery store? Meditate. Sitting in a boring meeting? Well, maybe don't meditate then, but you get the idea.

Herbal Supplements: If plants can grow in the harshest environments (looking at you, cacti!), they must have something going for them, right? Some women turn to herbal supplements like black cohosh, evening primrose oil, and St. John's Wort for relief from menopause symptoms. While the scientific jury is still out on some of these, others have shown promising results in research studies. Just remember to talk with your doctor before starting any new supplement regimen.

Acupuncture: Lastly, we've got acupuncture. This Chinese practice involves inserting tiny, thin needles into specific points on your body. If the thought of voluntarily getting poked with needles makes you wince, just remember that some people claim it can help with hot flashes and sleep problems. Plus, it gives you a great excuse to lie down for 20 minutes in the middle of the day.

These are just a handful of the many complementary therapies out there. The beauty of this approach is that you can mix and match therapies to find what works best for you. It's like being at a buffet, but instead of choosing between pasta and chicken, you're choosing between yoga and massage.

Who knew managing menopause could be so diverse?

Research on Complementary Therapies

Okay, so we've waxed lyrical about the range of complementary therapies and how they're like a buffet where you can mix and match to your heart's content. But let's get down to brass tacks. What does science say about all these treatments?

Now, keep in mind that we're entering a territory that has more plot twists than a soap opera. Not every therapy has been studied extensively, and among the ones that have, results often range from "Wow, this is better than sliced bread!" to "Hmm, this seems as effective as a chocolate teapot." So, let's dive in!

Yoga: In one study, women who participated in a yoga program reported a significant reduction in hot flashes and night sweats. But don't roll out your yoga mat just yet. Another study found no significant difference between a yoga group and a control group. The takeaway? More research is needed, but even if yoga doesn't directly impact your menopausal symptoms, it's still a great way to keep your body and mind fit.

Massage: While no large-scale studies have specifically targeted massage therapy for menopause symptoms, smaller studies and anecdotal evidence suggest that it may help reduce stress and improve sleep. And let's be real, who wouldn't feel better after a good rubdown?

Meditation: Researchers say this one's a keeper. Several studies have shown that mindfulness meditation can help reduce menopausal symptoms, particularly psychological ones like anxiety and depression. Some studies have even shown meditation to be as effective as CBT (cognitive-behavioral therapy) for improving sleep and reducing stress. Looks like those bald guys in orange robes are onto something!

Herbal Supplements: This is where things get a little spicy. Some studies suggest certain supplements might help with hot flashes. For example, black cohosh has shown some promise. But the studies are often small, and the results aren't always consistent. Plus, since supplements aren't regulated like medications, what you see might not always be what you get; if you are going to give any supplements a whirl, ensure you are buying from a reputable brand that stays away from additives. Ordering supplements can be like ordering a mystery box online; you never quite know what you're going to end up with!

Acupuncture: The research on acupuncture is like a roller coaster ride. One minute you're climbing up to a peak of promising results, and the next, you're plummeting into a valley of null findings. Some studies suggest acupuncture may be effective in reducing hot flashes, but other well-designed studies find no difference between real acupuncture and sham acupuncture. All in all, the evidence isn't robust enough to make a clear judgment.

The bottom line? Complementary therapies are as diverse as the research that supports them. It's important to approach these methods with an open mind but also with a healthy dose of skepticism. While they might not be the magic bullet for menopause symptoms, they can still play a role in your overall wellness strategy. After all, who wouldn't want more tools in their menopause management toolbox?

And remember, always check with your healthcare provider before starting any new treatment. They can help you weigh the potential benefits and risks, ensuring you make the best decision for your health.

KEY TAKEAWAYS

1. Complementary therapies offer a variety of approaches that can be integrated into your menopause management plan, from yoga and massage to meditation and herbal supplements.
2. Research on complementary therapies is as diverse as the therapies themselves. Some therapies show promise in reducing menopausal symptoms, while others need more robust research.
3. Always approach complementary therapies with an open mind and a healthy dose of skepticism. Effectiveness can vary widely from person to person.
4. It's essential to consult your healthcare provider before starting any new therapy. They can help you weigh the benefits and risks based on your specific health situation.
5. Despite the variability in effectiveness, complementary therapies can enhance your overall wellness strategy during menopause, offering more tools in your toolkit.

FINAL THOUGHTS

Embarking on the menopause journey might feel like you're wandering through a jungle without a map, but remember – you're not alone, and there are many paths you can take. Complementary therapies offer additional routes you can explore, adding to your repertoire of strategies to manage your menopause symptoms.

It's not about finding the one magic bullet but piecing together a puzzle that fits your unique needs. Embrace this period of change as an opportunity to discover new ways to support your well-being. After all, menopause isn't just a phase; it's an ongoing dance. And with the right tools and mindset, you can choreograph your routine to your own beat, turning this dance into a celebration of your resilience and strength.

Our next stop? A deep dive into the wide world of Hormone Replacement Therapy (HRT) and Bioidentical Hormone Therapy (BHT). They're more than just big words; they're potential game-changers for your menopause journey. See you on the other side!

A DEEP DIVE INTO HORMONE REPLACEMENT AND BIOIDENTICAL THERAPIES

Here's the thing about menopause: it's as subtle as a train wreck and about as comfortable as a cactus seat. And while the sisterhood of eternal hot flashes may sound like a cool club to be part of (spoiler alert: it's not), we're all seeking a little relief, right?

That's where our spotlight guests, Hormone Replacement Therapy (HRT) and Bioidentical Hormone Therapy (BHT), take the stage. They're no magic potion, but they're ready to roll up their sleeves and go toe-to-toe with some of your most bothersome menopause symptoms.

But hold onto your reading glasses – because it's not all smooth sailing. From potential side effects to controversies, I'm going to pop the hood on these therapies, giving you a front-row seat to the good, the bad, and the sweaty.

The goal? To arm you with all the knowledge you need to make the best decision.

HRT 101: WHAT'S THE DEAL WITH HORMONE REPLACEMENT THERAPY?

Let's dive deep into the molecular machinery of our bodies and explore Hormone Replacement Therapy or HRT. The principles of HRT are steeped in endocrinology, the study of hormones, and their breathtaking balancing act that keeps us ticking.

In essence, HRT is a medical strategy that supplements your body with hormones that start to wane as menopause sets in. Think of it as calling in reserves when your body's natural production lines of estrogen and progesterone slow down.

Estrogen, the diva hormone, is critical in regulating menstruation and reproductive processes in women. It's also linked to bone health, mood regulation, and even skin health, amongst others. Then there's progesterone, estrogen's lesser-known but equally hard-working sister, who's crucial in maintaining a healthy uterus, especially during pregnancy.

Menopause can cause these hormone levels to roller coaster before eventually dropping, leading to a slew of symptoms ranging from hot flashes and mood swings to sleep disturbances and bone density loss. HRT swoops in like a hormonal superhero, supplementing these hormones and helping to alleviate these symptoms.

But, like a well-curated playlist, HRT needs to be customized. It's not a one-size-fits-all treatment but is tailored based on individual symptoms, health history, and personal risk factors. Next, we'll delve into the types of HRT, each designed to meet specific needs in the symphony of menopause management.

TYPES OF HRT

When it comes to HRT, there's no one-size-fits-all. The wardrobe of options in HRT is quite extensive, ensuring that there's something to suit everyone's unique hormonal couture. Let's take a peek at some of these.

Estrogen Therapy

Let's introduce you to the solo artist of HRT – Estrogen Therapy.

As the name suggests, this therapy focuses on supplementing estrogen, the hormone that significantly dips during menopause. When your body hits the estrogen-pause button (yes, the pun was intended), you're left with symptoms like hot flashes and night sweats, and even vaginal dryness.

That's where estrogen therapy steps in, giving your body the much-needed estrogen boost. The therapy can be systemic, meaning it's available as a pill, patch, gel, spray, or injection and affects the entire body. However, it's typically reserved for women who've had a hysterectomy, as unopposed estrogen can up the ante on the risk of endometrial cancer. So, if you've still got your uterus, hold onto your horses because we've got another type of therapy for you.

Progesterone/Progestin Therapy

Say hello to Progesterone Therapy or its synthetic sibling, Progestin Therapy.

When estrogen is on solo duty, it can lead to an overgrowth of the endometrium (the lining of the uterus), which can increase the risk of endometrial cancer. To balance this, doctors prescribe progestin or progesterone. It's like estrogen's sidekick, ensuring the hormone doesn't go overboard.

Progesterone/progestin can be administered as a pill, intrauterine device (IUD), or in some cases, as a combination pill with estrogen. This is like a harmonious duet, balancing the effects of both hormones to manage menopause symptoms while protecting the uterus.

Combination Therapy (Estrogen and Progesterone)

Welcome to the power duet of menopause management: Combination Therapy. This consists of—you guessed it—both estrogen and progesterone. For women who still have their uterus intact, this therapy is a two-for-one deal. It helps alleviate menopausal symptoms while keeping the lining of the uterus in check.

This dynamic duo comes in several forms, like oral pills, skin patches, vaginal rings, or even injections. Depending on your health history, your doctor might recommend a continuous regimen (where you take both hormones daily) or a cyclic regimen (where you take estrogen daily and progesterone on certain days).

Local Estrogen Therapy

Local Estrogen Therapy is the covert operation of hormone replacement, focusing on specific problem areas. The treatment delivers a small dose of estrogen directly to the vaginal tissues, helping combat vaginal dryness, discomfort during sex, and urinary issues.

It's a bit like your local neighborhood watch, keeping an eye on a specific area rather than the whole town. The estrogen is delivered via a cream, tablet, or ring inserted into the vagina. It's a lower-dose alternative to systemic HRT and is ideal for women who primarily have vaginal menopause symptoms.

So, there you have it – a quick tour of the HRT boutique. It's a world filled with options tailored to meet individual needs. But remember, every woman's menopause journey is unique, and what works for one may not work for another. Always consult with your healthcare provider to identify the best therapeutic strategy for you.

MECHANISM OF HRT

It's one thing to know that HRT can help alleviate menopause symptoms, but it's quite another to understand how it does the job. It's a bit like magic—you know the rabbit comes out of the hat, but how does it get in there in the first place? Well, let's pull back the velvet curtain and take a closer look at the enchanting world of HRT.

How These Hormones Work to Relieve Menopause Symptoms

Let's start with the obvious: how do these hormones actually relieve the symptoms of menopause? In essence, it's like a fill-the-gap solution.

As we mentioned before, menopause is basically your body's way of saying, "Okay, we're done with the baby-making phase, let's move on to something new." And just like any other major life transition (think midlife crisis or teenage angst), it comes with its own set of issues. The main one being your body going on a hormone strike.

In the case of menopause, your ovaries, those faithful little hormone factories, decide to retire early. They downsize their production of estrogen and progesterone—two hormones that have been calling the shots in your body since puberty. The result? A full-blown hormone revolt, with symptoms

ranging from hot flashes and mood swings to sleep disturbances and vaginal dryness.

But fret not, for HRT plays the role of a skilled diplomat in
this hormonal conflict. By supplementing the body with doses
of estrogen and/or progesterone, HRT restores the hormonal
balance, thereby helping to alleviate the symptoms of
menopause. Think of it like quelling a riot by giving the
protesters what they want—peace and quiet return, and you
can go about your day without being drenched in sweat or
snapping at your partner for breathing too loudly.

The Role of Estrogen and Progesterone in the Body

Now, before we delve deeper into how HRT works its magic,
let's take a moment to appreciate the star performers of our
show - estrogen and progesterone. These hormones are the yin
and yang of female reproductive health, each with its own set
of crucial responsibilities.

Starting with the queen bee, estrogen. This hormone is like
the director of a blockbuster movie - it has a hand in everything. From kickstarting puberty and developing secondary
sexual characteristics to regulating menstrual cycles and maintaining pregnancy, estrogen plays a vital role. But that's not all.
It also influences bone health, heart health, mood, and even
skin health. It's like the multitasker we all aspire to be.

Next up is progesterone, the unsung hero. While it might not
bask in the limelight as much as estrogen, it's just as important. Progesterone is chiefly responsible for preparing the
uterus for pregnancy after ovulation, maintaining pregnancy,
and regulating the menstrual cycle. It's the behind-the-scenes
worker who ensures everything runs smoothly.

So, when the production of these hormones drops during
menopause, your body kind of misses them (understandably

so!). It's like going from a full orchestra to a lone violinist - the symphony just isn't the same. And that's where HRT steps in, tuning the instruments and getting the band back together to play the harmonious symphony of well-being once more.

But remember, just like every orchestra needs a good conductor, your HRT journey needs a good healthcare provider. It's crucial to have an expert guide who can customize the therapy to your needs, monitor the effects, and make necessary adjustments. After all, we all want our menopausal symphony to be a chart-topping hit, right?

BENEFITS OF HRT

So far, we've talked about how HRT steps up to the plate when our body decides to put a halt to its hormone production. It's like having a pinch-hitter in a baseball game - and if you're anything like me and sports metaphors go right over your head, let's just say it's a good thing. But what are the tangible benefits of HRT? What can you, as a menopausal woman, expect from it? The answers are as satisfying as a perfect chocolate chip cookie – comforting, delightful, and just what you need.

Relief from Hot Flashes and Night Sweats

Imagine sitting in a business meeting or enjoying a romantic dinner when a rogue wave of heat washes over you. Suddenly, you're as sweaty as a marathoner, but all you've done is pass the salt! Enter hot flashes - uninvited guests at the party of menopause. And their annoying cousin, night sweats, ensures you don't even get respite in your dreams.

The good news is HRT can be your reliable bouncer, showing these party crashers the door. Estrogen, in particular, has been shown to significantly reduce the frequency and intensity of hot flashes and night sweats. It's like having a personal body-guard against these intrusive symptoms, making sure your days (and nights) go undisturbed. Ah, sweet relief!

Improvement of Vaginal Symptoms

Then there are the hush-hush issues, the ones we often hesitate to discuss – vaginal dryness, itching, burning, and discomfort during sex. No, you're not alone, and no, you don't have to endure it in silence.

HRT is like that friend who rushes to your side with a comforting arm around your shoulders (or in this case, your lady parts). Estrogen therapy, particularly local estrogen therapy, can revitalize the vaginal tissues by increasing blood flow and elasticity while also boosting natural lubrication. You see, it's not all doom and gloom in the menopause town. There's help, there's support, and there's HRT.

Protection Against Bone Loss and Fracture

Last but not least, let's talk bones. Our skeletal system, the very framework that holds us up, is also at the mercy of declining estrogen levels during menopause. Lower levels of estrogen can lead to decreased bone density, resulting in a higher risk of fractures. It's like your internal scaffolding losing its stability - not an ideal scenario.

But guess who's donned the superhero cape again? That's right, HRT! Hormone replacement therapy, especially with estrogen, can slow down bone loss and decrease the risk of fractures. It's like having your personal construction crew working tirelessly to maintain your infrastructure. Not all heroes wear capes; some just balance hormones!

So, as you can see, the benefits of HRT are pretty impressive. But it's also important to remember that, like any therapy,

HRT is not one-size-fits-all. It's a journey that needs to be tailored to your body, your symptoms, and your health history. So, don't shy away from having open, detailed discussions with your healthcare provider. After all, they're the co-pilot on your menopause journey!

RISKS AND SIDE EFFECTS OF HRT

Let's pull back the curtain on the lesser-glamorous side of HRT, the risk, and the side effects. It's like planning a dream vacation - you focus on the exciting bits: the exotic locales, the delicious food, the Instagram-worthy moments. But you also need to consider the potential hiccups: lost luggage, food poisoning, getting photobombed by a pigeon. Similarly, while HRT comes with its package of benefits, it also carries certain risks and side effects. Remember, knowledge is power - even when it's not particularly cheery.

Short-Term Side Effects

Just like how your favorite chocolate bar comes with the not-so-sweet calories, HRT may come with some short-term side effects. These are typically mild and transient, kind of like those pesky fruit flies in summer. They're annoying, but they don't stick around for long.

Bloating: It's like your body decided to throw a surprise balloon party in your belly. But fear not, this tends to subside as your body adjusts to the therapy. Drinking plenty of water, eating a high-fiber diet, and regular exercise can help.

Breast Tenderness: You might feel like your girls are going through a moody teenager phase—sensitive, tender, and a bit painful. Again, this tends to improve over time, but if it doesn't, have a chat with your doctor.

Mood Swings: If you're riding an emotional roller-coaster, hormones could be the amusement park operators. They influence your brain chemistry and can lead to mood swings. Regular exercise, a healthy diet, and good sleep can be your stabilizers.

Nausea: Some people might experience a bit of queasiness, like having motion sickness, without setting foot in a vehicle. Taking your HRT with food can help keep your stomach settled.

Long-Term Risks

Now for the long-term risks. These are like the lurking trolls under the bridge - rarer but more serious. The relationship between HRT and these conditions is complex, kind of like trying to untangle a necklace chain – tricky and needing careful handling.

Heart Disease: Early initiation of HRT (around the time of menopause) may have a protective effect on the heart. But for older women or those starting HRT more than 10-20 years after menopause, the story can be different. It's like trying to start a marathon after everyone else has crossed the halfway point – not ideal.

Stroke and Blood Clots: HRT, especially oral estrogen, can increase the risk of blood clots and stroke. Think of these as unwanted traffic jams in your body's highways – something we want to avoid.

Breast Cancer: The relationship between HRT and breast cancer is nuanced. Estrogen-only therapy does not appear to increase breast cancer risk significantly, but combined estrogen-progestin therapy might after several years of use. So, it's important to have an open, detailed discussion with your doctor to weigh the pros and cons based on your personal risk profile.

Remember, everyone's body is unique and will respond differently to HRT. The key is to have an ongoing conversation with your doctor, one where you openly discuss your symptoms, concerns, and lifestyle. Together, you can create a tailored treatment plan that best fits you, like finding that perfect pair of jeans – it takes some trial and error, but it's worth it!

WHO CAN AND CAN NOT USE HRT

So, is HRT a one-size-fits-all miracle for every woman riding the menopause roller coaster? Well, not quite. Like that 'one size fits all' label on a dress that just doesn't cut it, eligibility for HRT isn't universal. Let's delve into the factors that make a difference.

Medical History Factors That Influence HRT Suitability

Consider your medical history as your body's diary - an account of past incidents that shape your present and future health decisions. Just as you'd refer back to previous diary entries before meeting an old friend, your doctor will consider your medical history when discussing HRT.

Here are some key 'entries' that might pop up:

Previous Breast or Endometrial Cancer: If you've had a close encounter with these cancers, HRT might not be the best fit. It's like a reunion with an ex-flame who's bad news - best to keep your distance.

Liver Disease: If your liver isn't doing its detox gig well due to disease, HRT might add to its burden. Like adding another task to an already overflowing to-do list.

History of Blood Clots or Stroke: Got a history of blood clots or stroke? Oral HRT could be like throwing oil onto a sputtering fire. However, transdermal methods might still be an option.

Heart Disease: Recent heart disease or heart attack might push HRT into the 'no-go' zone. Like being told to avoid sweets when you've just been diagnosed with diabetes.

Uncontrolled High Blood Pressure: If your blood pressure is dancing the tango on the higher end, your doctor might want to get that under control before considering HRT. Like securing your oxygen mask first before assisting others.

Age Considerations

Your age also plays a pivotal role in determining HRT suitability. HRT for younger women, typically those in their early 50s or within 10 years of menopause onset, has a more favorable benefit-risk profile. It's like getting a front-row seat at a concert - better view, better experience. However, starting HRT later (typically beyond 60 or 10-20 years after menopause) may increase certain risks.

ALTERNATIVES TO HRT

Let's say HRT, and you didn't exactly match on a medical Tinder. Or perhaps you've tried it and found it wasn't your cup of herbal tea. Fear not, my friend! We have a few alternative headliners ready to take the stage.

Non-Hormonal Prescription Medications

Certain antidepressants, blood pressure medications, and even anti-seizure drugs have been found to help with hot flashes. It's like finding out your smartphone also works as a bottle opener - not its main gig, but handy nonetheless!

Lifestyle Changes

Ain't nothing like a good ol' lifestyle makeover! Small changes can bring big impacts.

Regular Exercise: Breaking a sweat can help reduce hot flashes and improve sleep. Plus, it's a ticket to the feel-good endorphins party!

Healthy Diet: Fueling your body with a balanced diet helps manage weight and keeps your heart happy. It's like giving your body the premium fuel it deserves.

Reduced Caffeine and Alcohol: These might trigger hot flashes and affect sleep. Consider them the party crashers of menopause.

Quit Smoking: Cigarette smoking can increase hot flashes and bring about earlier menopause. Need another reason to break up with this toxic relationship?

Natural Remedies

For those preferring the scenic route, natural remedies might appeal.

Soy and Black Cohosh: Some research suggests they might help with mild hot flashes. But do check with your doc first, as they can interact with other medications.

Yoga and Acupuncture: These have shown promise in managing some menopause symptoms. It's like a spa day for your hormones!

Remember, just because HRT isn't your match, doesn't mean you're left to brave menopause alone. There's a plethora of options out there, and one (or a combination) could be your perfect fit. It might take some trial and error, but hang in there champ! Together, we've got this!

BIOIDENTICAL HORMONE THERAPY: THE 'NATURAL' PATH THROUGH MENOPAUSE

We've been through the HRT express, now let's switch gears and ride down the scenic route of Bioidentical Hormone Therapy, or BHT for short. No, it's not a fancy new hipster sandwich on the menu of your local cafe, but it is something that's gaining popularity among menopausal women faster than cat videos on the internet.

What is Bioidentical Hormone Therapy

Bioidentical Hormone Therapy sounds like something straight out of a sci-fi movie, doesn't it? But let's break it down in simple terms. 'Bio,' meaning life, and 'identical,' meaning, well, identical, essentially refers to hormones that are molecularly identical to those produced by your own body. In other words, these hormones are as close as you can get to the real thing without robbing your younger self.

Think of it this way: BHT is like hiring an Elvis impersonator for your birthday party. They might not be the real King, but boy, can they bring the house down with a riveting rendition of "Jailhouse Rock"!

Purpose and Use in Treating Menopause Symptoms

The spotlight on bioidentical hormones has grown brighter in recent years, and they're no longer the understudy in the grand play of menopause management. Why? Well, as your body's hormone production wanes during menopause (yes, they're taking an unannounced sabbatical), bioidentical hormones step in to keep the show running smoothly.

Similar to the way HRT replenishes your body with hormones, BHT does the same, but with a little more customization. It's like the difference between off-the-rack clothing and tailored-to-fit couture. These hormones can be specifically designed to match your body's unique needs.

BHT helps manage those pesky menopausal symptoms like hot flashes, night sweats, mood changes, memory problems, weight gain, sleep issues, loss of interest in sex, or low energy. It's like having a super-nanny swooping in, Mary Poppins-style, to calm the chaos in the hormonal household of your body.

From creams and gels to patches, pills, pellet therapy, and injections, bioidentical hormones come in various forms, giving you options. It's like a buffet table of relief, where you can choose the serving method that suits you best!

In a nutshell, BHT is all about managing menopause symptoms by introducing hormones that your body recognizes as its own, ensuring a smooth transition during this new phase of life. It's the doppelgänger of your own hormones, helping maintain the equilibrium and harmony in your body.

BIOIDENTICAL VS. SYNTHETIC HORMONES

Get ready because we're about to embark on a face-off of epic proportions - bioidentical hormones versus synthetic hormones. This isn't Godzilla versus King Kong, but it's just as monumental in the world of menopause.

The Difference in Molecular Structure

If hormones were twins, bioidentical hormones would be the identical twin while synthetic hormones would be the fraternal one. They're both family, but one's an exact copy while the other is, well, close but not quite.

Bioidentical hormones have the same molecular structure as the hormones naturally produced by your body. That's like comparing two copies of the Mona Lisa. If you're not a seasoned art critic (or even if you are), you'll find it hard to tell them apart.

On the other hand, synthetic hormones, while designed to mimic the effects of natural hormones, aren't exactly the same. They're like the cover version of your favorite song. The words and melody are familiar, but the voice is different, and sometimes, the notes don't hit quite right.

Body's Reception and Usage of Both

Now, let's chat about how your body receives these two types of hormones. You can think of your body as an exclusive club. Bioidentical hormones are on the VIP list, so they breeze through the velvet ropes, get recognized by the bouncer (your body's hormone receptors), and start partying right away (benefiting your body).

Synthetic hormones, however, might have a bit more trouble at the door. They're like your cousin's friend's boyfriend who claims he's on the list. The bouncer squints at them, sees they're not an exact match to the club's preference, but often lets them in anyway. Once inside, they can still get the party going (provide relief for menopausal symptoms), but it's a bit of a different vibe (they may work differently and have different side effects than bioidentical hormones).

The main thing to remember is that the body can utilize both types of hormones, but the experience may vary due to the differences in their molecular structures. It's like choosing between a home-cooked meal and fast food. Both will feed you, but the home-cooked meal might feel a little more like, well, home. That being said, some bodies prefer fast food, and that's okay too!

TYPES OF BIOIDENTICAL HORMONES

Bioidentical hormones come in many different varieties, like flavors of your favorite ice cream. However, the two superstars in our menopausal journey are Bioidentical Estrogen and Bioidentical Progesterone. Let's get to know these two a bit better.

Bioidentical Estrogen

Consider Bioidentical Estrogen as the cherry on top of your menopausal sundae. It's meant to replicate the natural estrogen that your body produces (or rather, used to produce) to keep everything running smoothly. Just as a cherry completes your sundae, bioidentical estrogen restores some harmony to your system by alleviating those pesky hot flashes and safeguarding your bones against osteoporosis.

Bioidentical Progesterone

Next up, we have Bioidentical Progesterone, the unsung hero in this hormonal saga. It may not have the same star power as estrogen but don't underestimate its importance. It's a vital component for those who still have a uterus because it helps protect the lining of your uterus from becoming too thick – something that can lead to complications.

ADMINISTRATION OF BIOIDENTICAL HORMONE THERAPY

Now, how do we introduce these friendly bioidentical hormones into your body, you may wonder? Let's explore some of the common delivery methods.

Pills

Popping a pill is probably the most traditional way of getting your daily dose of bioidentical hormones. It's as simple as swigging it down with a glass of water or, if you're feeling cheeky, your favorite wine (though your doctor might frown upon this). Pills are convenient, but they do require a pit stop in the liver before the hormones can get to work, which may influence their effectiveness.

Patches

For those of you who aren't fans of swallowing pills, consider patches. Think of them as little hormone couriers that deliver your bioidentical hormone dosage through your skin and directly into your bloodstream. It's like having your very own hormone concierge service!

Topical Creams

A bit of cream anyone? No, I'm not talking about dessert. Bioidentical hormones can also come in topical creams or gels that you apply to your skin. Think of it as a moisturizer with a menopause-defying bonus.

Vaginal Suppositories

Next, we have vaginal suppositories. This method might sound a bit intimidating, but they're great for targeting local symptoms like dryness or irritation. Think of them as your personal firefighters, ready to douse the flame of any vaginal discomfort.

Pellet Therapy

Lastly, for some women, hormone pellet therapy may be the way to go. Its 2-3 small pellets about the size of a grain of rice are inserted beneath the skin into the fatty tissue of the hip, and the pure hormone is delivered gradually, directly into the bloodstream. This is the easy fire-and-forget method.

BENEFITS OF BIOIDENTICAL HORMONE THERAPY

Now that we've journeyed through the land of bioidentical hormone types and delivery methods let's dive into the perks of these little molecular powerhouses. Just like Hormone Replacement Therapy (HRT), bioidentical hormones strive to alleviate those hot flashes that can turn you into a human torch, those bone-depleting monsters (hello osteoporosis!), and the parade of other menopausal symptoms that leave you wondering, "Who hijacked my body?"

The standout feature of bioidentical hormones, however, is their star performance of being more like your body's natural hormones. This means that your body rolls out the red carpet for them, celebrating their close resemblance to your native hormones. As a result, many women report experiencing fewer side effects than with traditional HRT. Sounds like a pretty sweet deal, right?

But remember, just as in any celebrity saga, everything that glitters isn't always gold.

RISKS AND SIDE EFFECTS OF BIOIDENTICAL HORMONE THERAPY

Bioidentical hormones may be the new kids on the block in the world of menopause treatment, but they're not without controversy. Picture a new actor in a long-running TV series: exciting but potentially disruptive. That's exactly what's happening in the scientific community surrounding these substances.

One of the key controversies revolves around the lack of long-term research. Although bioidentical hormones have shown promise, the lack of long-term studies leaves many questions unanswered. Think of it as a season finale with a nail-biting cliffhanger. We're all waiting for the next season to drop so we can find out what happens next.

To make matters more challenging, many experts believe that bioidentical hormones may come with the same risks as traditional HRT. This includes potential increased risks for heart disease, stroke, blood clots, and breast cancer. It's like binge-watching your favorite thriller and realizing the villain could be any one of the characters.

So, while we'd all love for bioidentical hormones to be the simple, side-effect-free solution to our menopause woes, the reality is a bit more complicated. As with any treatment, it's crucial to have a frank conversation with your healthcare provider about potential risks and benefits.

WHO CAN AND CANNOT USE BIOIDENTICAL HORMONE THERAPY

Alright, we've talked the talk about bioidentical hormones, but now it's time to walk the walk. Or, more specifically, let's figure out who gets an invitation to this hormone party and who might want to RSVP with a polite "No, thank you."

Generally, the ideal candidates for bioidentical hormone therapy (BHT) aren't that different from those who might benefit from HRT. If menopause has decided to crash your life's party like an uninvited guest, making you all hot and bothered (literally), then you might be a candidate for BHT.

But, and this is a big "but", BHT may not be the best option for everyone. Just like how not everyone can pull off neon green eyeshadow (and if you can, more power to you!), not every woman can or should use bioidentical hormones. The decision to use BHT isn't as simple as picking out an outfit for a casual Friday.

In particular, women with a history of breast cancer, ovarian cancer, endometrial cancer, blood clots, stroke, or heart disease might need to steer clear from both HRT and BHT. Also, if you're a smoker or over 60, caution is advised. Always discuss your personal health history and risks with your healthcare provider to make sure you're making the safest and most effective choice for you. And if your physician isn't asking about these factors, that's like a hairdresser not asking about your hair type before giving you a perm – not okay!

CUSTOM-COMPOUNDED BIOIDENTICAL HORMONES: THE NEW KIDS ON THE BLOCK

Now that we've navigated the eligibility maze let's move onto a hot topic: custom-compounded bioidentical hormones. It sounds fancy, right? But what does it really mean?

"Custom compounded" refers to the practice of customizing a patient's hormone mix based on their unique needs. Imagine a bespoke suit, but it's your hormone therapy tailored to you. Pretty cool, huh?

But hold your horses because there's some controversy circling this custom couture hormone therapy. The main point of contention lies in the lack of oversight. These custom concoctions are not FDA-approved, which means they've not undergone rigorous testing for safety, efficacy, or consistency. It's kind of like buying a designer dress from a sketchy online site that doesn't offer returns - it might work out, but it might also be a disaster.

The FDA has been pretty vocal about this issue, issuing warnings about the potential risks of compounded BHT. It's like the stern parent chiding you not to accept candy from strangers - they're just looking out for your best interest. These risks might include inconsistent doses, contaminants, or undisclosed side effects.

KEY TAKEAWAYS

1. HRT and BHT can help mitigate menopausal symptoms by replenishing diminishing hormone levels.
2. There are diverse forms of HRT and BHT - pills, patches, creams, and suppositories, each tailored to individual needs.
3. Despite their benefits, both therapies carry potential short-term side effects and long-term risks.
4. Not everyone is a candidate for these therapies. Medical history and age greatly influence suitability.
5. Bioidentical Hormone Therapy, while promising, lacks extensive long-term research and is surrounded by controversy, especially with custom compounded hormones.

FINAL THOUGHTS

And there we have it, ladies and gents - your crash course in the world of Hormone Replacement Therapy and Bioidentical Hormone Therapy. Menopause may feel like you've been thrown into the deep end, but with tools like HRT and BHT, you've got a couple of nifty lifebuoys to help keep you afloat.

Remember, everyone's menopause journey is unique. These therapies are not a magic bullet, but they can be part of a broader strategy to manage your menopausal symptoms. The key is to have open, honest conversations with your healthcare provider to find a treatment plan tailored to your needs.

Navigating menopause may seem like sailing in uncharted waters. But equipped with knowledge, humor, and a pinch of patience, you'll be able to ride the waves with grace. After all, as we've come to learn, menopause is not the end of the road. It's meCustom-Compoundedyour life's journey. So why not make it a memorable one?

Now, let's tune into our next chapter, "Can modern medicine help me?" We'll explore the role of the good old doc in your menopause journey, including what to expect, what to ask, and how to navigate the medical waters. Because even in the face of menopause, knowledge is power, and you're the captain of your ship.

CAN MODERN MEDICINE ALLEVIATE MENOPAUSE SYMPTOMS?

Now that we've journeyed through the whats, whys, and hows of menopause in previous chapters, it's time to explore the world of modern medicine. We're talking about the white-coated, lab-dwelling, cutting-edge stuff that's saving lives and making headlines.

So you're facing the meno-storm, wondering, "How can I possibly navigate this tempest?" Well, the answer could lie in the very place where science and symptoms intersect: the realm of modern medicine.

Before we dive any deeper, it's vital to remember this key point: menopause is not an illness. It's as natural as sunrise and sunset, as common as the changing of the seasons. It's a part of life, a transition every woman goes through. So why are we talking about medicine at all, you might wonder? Well, while menopause itself doesn't need a cure, some of its symptoms can be like uninvited party crashers, disrupting your life when you least expect it. And that's where modern medicine comes in.

Just like you might take an aspirin to soothe a headache or antihistamines to curb those pesky allergy symptoms, modern medicine offers ways to manage the sometimes challenging symptoms of menopause. They're not eradicating menopause (and nor should they), but they can help you navigate this natural transition with more ease and comfort.

Remember that while the information in this chapter could be a life-saver (literally), it should never replace professional medical advice. I'm here to offer insights and options, but your healthcare provider should always be your first port of call when it comes to managing your symptoms. Now, onto the good stuff!

DIAGNOSING MENOPAUSE

Diagnosing menopause is a bit like spotting a bear in the wild. You may have never seen a bear before, but when one saunters across your path, you'd probably go, "Yup, that's a bear." Much like our bear analogy, menopause doesn't often require Sherlock Holmes-level detective work. Its signs and symptoms can be so distinct that most women can recognize it themselves. But remember, a bear sighting is one thing; knowing how to navigate around the bear is quite another.

When to Consult a Doctor

It's not like you'd stroll through the storm without an umbrella, right? Menopause, with its battalion of changes, can sometimes feel like a sudden downpour. You may experience a range of symptoms like hot flashes, irregular periods, or the not-so-enjoyable midnight sweat-a-thons. These are the menopausal equivalent of thunderclaps. And when these thunderclaps echo in your life, it's time to ring up your healthcare provider.

Sure, menopause is a natural part of life, like growing old or becoming obsessed with gardening. But just because it's natural doesn't mean you should "grin and bear it." If something's making you uncomfortable or is out of your ordinary, it's worth discussing with a professional.

You see, your doctor is more than a lab coat and stethoscope. They're your teammate, your co-pilot through the turbulence of menopause. They ought to be equipped to decode your body's intricate changes and help you manage any accompanying discomforts. However, not every physician possesses this knowledge or understanding. It might take you a few trials before you find the right one. But don't give up. Keep seeking until you find that health professional who doesn't just listen but truly hears and understands you.

It's also important to remember that while menopause is universal, how it plays out can be as unique as your fingerprint. Some of us might breeze through it, while others may feel like they're juggling flaming torches on a unicycle. Your healthcare provider can help you understand your unique symptoms and what they mean for you.

So, when should you definitely pick up the phone? If your periods are so heavy they interfere with your daily activities, if they come very close together, or if you experience spotting between periods or following sex, these are crucial times to seek advice. And hey, even if your questions might seem small or your symptoms minor, don't hesitate to dial that number. When it comes to your health, there's no such thing as a silly question. After all, you wouldn't ignore a warning light on your car's dashboard, would you?

Navigating menopause isn't about suffering in silence or getting lost in the wild woods of internet searches. It's about having an open line of communication with your doctor and ensuring that your journey through this transition is as smooth and comfortable as possible. So, pick up the phone, schedule that appointment, and take that step towards understanding and managing your menopause.

Now, you might be wondering what happens during a typical menopause evaluation. Well, your doctor won't wave a magic wand or use a crystal ball (if they do, you may want to consider switching doctors). Instead, they'll usually have a chat with you about your symptoms, review your medical history, and may carry out a physical examination. This isn't the Spanish Inquisition – it's just a straightforward, no-frills assessment.

Role of FSH Levels

Let's dive into the alphabet soup of menopause diagnosis: FSH. No, it's not the name of a fancy, avant-garde artist or a rare bird species. FSH, or Follicle Stimulating Hormone, plays a starring role in our bodies' reproductive narratives, and it can give some valuable insights into the onset of menopause.

FSH is the biological maestro that orchestrates the monthly cycle of egg production in women. When it waves its metaphorical baton, the ovarian follicles respond, gearing up for the potential of pregnancy each month. But as menopause begins to loom, your ovaries start to retire from their egg-releasing gig, much like a tired rock star might hang up their electric guitar.

This exit from the reproductive stage doesn't go unnoticed. Your body, ever the persistent stage manager, tries to coax a performance out of the ovaries by cranking up the FSH levels - it's a bit like turning up the volume on your radio when your favorite song comes on. Your body is just trying to get your ovaries to tune into the same station.

This increase in FSH level can be a useful pointer that menopause is en route. But it's not quite as simple as just taking a snapshot of your FSH levels at one moment in time. Hormone levels can fluctuate, and FSH is no exception to this rule. A single elevated FSH level might be like a false alarm, an overly eager party guest who shows up while you're still in your bathrobe. This is why doctors often test FSH levels at different times to ensure they're not being led astray by one unusual result.

It's also important to remember that FSH is not the be-all and end-all marker of menopause. It's more like a piece of a complex jigsaw puzzle. Other factors come into play, like your age, symptoms, and menstrual history. It's by piecing these elements together that your healthcare provider can get a clear picture of where you are on your menopause journey.

So there you have it! FSH levels - another crucial character in the captivating drama of menopause. It might not have the most lines or the catchiest name, but it sure does play a pivotal role in our understanding of this unique life transition. After all, who doesn't love a good behind-the-scenes look?

Limitations of Over-the-Counter Home Tests

For the do-it-yourself fans, the concept of an over-the-counter menopause test might seem like a no-brainer. It's simple: buy a kit, take it home, pee on a stick, and voila! You've got your answers. Or do you? These tests work by detecting levels of FSH in your urine, a bit like how a home pregnancy test hunts down pregnancy hormones. And while this might sound like a one-stop solution to your menopause questions, it's important to understand their limitations.

Just as no two women experience menopause in the exact same way, FSH levels can fluctuate and are as unpredictable as a cliffhanger on a TV drama series. They can rise and fall throughout your menstrual cycle, like the tides of the ocean, making it challenging to get a precise reading at any one time. The elevated FSH level detected by a home test on one day might recede the next. So, these tests can sometimes create more questions than they answer.

Furthermore, while these home tests can indicate elevated FSH levels, they're a bit like an unfinished book – they don't give you the full story or the intricate plot details. They might provide a general indication, an initial sketch, but they're not as reliable or comprehensive as a lab test or an assessment from your healthcare provider, who has the full library of your health history and symptoms at hand.

Consider these over-the-counter tests as part of a larger tool-box. They can be a useful starting point, a prelude to the main act if you will. But remember, they shouldn't be used in isolation to make decisions about your health or treatment. It's a bit like trying to make a soufflé with just an egg – you're going to need a few more ingredients for success.

Lastly, if you're worried about cost, think about this: is it worth paying for a test that might not give you the complete, accurate information you need? Sometimes, the best course of action is to invest in a consultation with your healthcare provider, who can guide you based on a broad understanding of menopause and your specific circumstances.

So, by all means, explore the world of over-the-counter tests if you wish. But remember, they're not the magical crystal ball that can reveal the full panorama of your menopause status. When it comes to understanding menopause, it seems there really isn't a shortcut. But hey, who doesn't enjoy a bit of a scenic route?

THE PERSONALIZED CARE APPROACH

Embarking on the menopause journey is akin to stepping onto a dance floor where the music changes tempo without warning. Everyone has their unique dance style to keep up with these shifts. This is precisely why menopause care cannot, and should not, be a cookie-cutter approach.

The 'one-size-fits-all' method may work for adjustable baseball caps or universal smartphone chargers, but when it comes to managing the multifaceted experience of menopause, it simply falls short.

Importance of Individualized Treatment Plans

If you've ever had a coffee order that sounded more like a secret code - "Double-shot mocha latte with oat milk, 94 degrees, no foam, a sprinkle of cinnamon and served in a mug, not a cup" – then you'll appreciate the need for personalization. And this principle doesn't stop at coffee. When it comes to managing menopause, we're not looking for a one-size-fits-all cap. We want that tailor-made, fits-like-a-glove treatment plan.

Each woman's experience is unique. Your friend might've sailed through menopause on a gentle breeze while you feel like you're navigating a tempest. That's because our bodies aren't cookie-cutter models. Each one has a unique combination of genetics, lifestyle factors, health history, and more. What works wonders for one woman might do zilch for another.

This is where individualized treatment plans strut onto the stage. These plans aren't plucked out of thin air; they're designed after a careful review of your symptoms, history, and preferences. Picture a tailor taking your measurements, ensuring each stitch and seam matches your contours. That's what a healthcare provider does with an individualized treatment plan – ensuring the approach fits your specific needs, making the journey of menopause more like a steady stroll rather than an uphill slog.

Keeping a Symptom Diary/Journal: Linking Mood Swings and Changes

Now, let's talk about the mood swing conundrum. If you've ever felt as changeable as a chameleon in a tie-dye factory during your menopausal transition, know that you're not alone. One moment you're joyfully singing in the shower; the next, you're contemplating the existential dread of the forgotten conditioner. Menopause can sometimes feel like an emotional roller coaster, but how can we pin down these mood swings and, more importantly, manage them?

Enter the power of the symptom diary/journal! As we talked about all the way back in Chapter 2, I've created your very own Menopause Journal/Diary titled *"Menopause Makeover: A Guided Journal for Transformation."* Available on Amazon, this journal is more than just a tracking tool. It's a companion that walks with you through your menopause journey and all the things you may experience. You might have thought diaries were just for adolescent angst and doodles of your crush. Still, it turns out they can be a powerful tool in understanding and managing your menopausal symptoms.

So, what does keeping a symptom diary involve? Here are some tips:

Noting Down Symptoms: Write down any physical or emotional symptoms you experience and when they occur. You might notice some patterns, like an increase in irritability around the time you usually experience hot flashes.

Logging Food and Beverage Intake: Some women find certain foods or drinks trigger their hot flashes or mood swings. By keeping a log, you might spot links between what you consume and how you feel.

Recording Sleep Patterns: Insufficient sleep can amplify emotional responses. By noting down your sleep patterns, you might find a correlation between poor sleep and increased mood swings.

Tracking Exercise: Physical activity has been shown to improve mood and decrease symptoms like hot flashes. Monitor your exercise routine and any changes in symptoms that follow.

The benefits of a symptom diary stretch beyond mood management. It can help you and your healthcare provider understand your unique experience with menopause and develop a more tailored treatment approach. So grab a pen, snag a notebook of your own or a ready-made version, and let the power of observation (and a little note-taking) help you unlock the mysteries of your mood swings. It's like being your own detective but without the ominous trench coat and foggy alleyways.

Remember, managing menopause isn't about "just dealing with it" - it's about understanding your body's changes, finding effective coping strategies, and embracing this new chapter in your life with knowledge, support, and perhaps a dash of humor. Because who said menopause has to be all hot flashes and no fun?

THE OB-GYN'S ROLE IN CARE

As the story of menopause unfolds, your OB-GYN becomes a critical character. This medical professional is your trusted guide and ally, helping you understand the twists and turns of your own unique narrative.

Importance of Regular Consultations

Staying connected with your OB-GYN during menopause isn't just about addressing immediate health concerns—it's about ongoing, proactive management. Regular check-ups provide a platform to discuss any new or shifting symptoms, track changes in your menstrual cycle, and enable early detection and treatment of any health issues related to menopause. So yes, reaching out to your OB-GYN should be a recurring event in your calendar.

Consider these check-ups as your lifeline to better health during menopause. During these visits, your doctor can closely monitor your symptoms and adjust your treatment plan, as needed, to help you better manage these symptoms. They can offer recommendations on lifestyle changes, hormone therapy, or other treatments that can help mitigate the effects of menopause. They're also a great time to discuss any mental or emotional changes you've been experiencing, as mood swings and depression can often accompany menopause.

Regular visits also allow your doctor to conduct necessary health screenings that are crucial during menopause. For example, due to the decrease in estrogen levels, post-menopausal women are at a higher risk of osteoporosis. Timely bone density tests can detect early signs of this condition, and appropriate measures can be taken to protect your bone health.

Understanding Changes and Adapting to Them with Professional Guidance

The process of menopause is like navigating a maze—you know there's an exit, but the path is unpredictable. Your OB-GYN serves as your guide, helping to illuminate the way through the labyrinth of hormonal fluctuations and the changes they trigger in your body. They're there to help you understand what to expect, why certain changes occur, and how to manage them. Plus, they assist you in modifying your care plan as needed, ensuring you're equipped with the best strategies for your journey.

For instance, you might experience weight gain during menopause due to the change in hormones and metabolism. Your OB-GYN can provide insights into why this is happening and offer practical tips for managing it, like changes in diet or exercise regimen. They can also explain how hormonal changes can affect your skin, hair, and overall appearance and guide you to appropriate solutions.

Sleep disturbances and hot flashes are two very common symptoms of menopause. Instead of leaving you to deal with these on your own, your OB-GYN can provide proven techniques to manage these symptoms. This might include everything from hormone therapy to simple changes in your sleep environment.

Menopause can also impact your sexual health. The decrease in estrogen levels can lead to vaginal dryness, making intercourse uncomfortable. Your OB-GYN can suggest safe and effective treatments to counter these issues and ensure a healthy and satisfying sex life during menopause.

The takeaway here is that the journey through menopause is deeply personal, with each woman's experience differing from the next. There's no one-size-fits-all approach, and having the right and a trusted OB-GYN on your side can make all the difference in successfully navigating this phase of life.

DETERMINING MENOPAUSE STAGE THROUGH BLOOD TESTS

Have you ever tried to find out how much gas is left in a propane tank by lifting it? It's not an exact science, is it? You heft the thing, swish it around a bit, and then make your best guess. Well, trying to figure out where you are in the menopause journey without proper testing can feel just as vague. Luckily, science has provided us with something a tad more accurate than the old lift-and-guess. Enter blood tests!

Process and Purpose

Blood tests during menopause are a valuable tool to assess the levels of certain hormones in your body, specifically FSH and estradiol.

Remember our old friend FSH (Follicle Stimulating Hormone)? Its levels increase as the number of eggs in your ovaries decreases. So, a higher level of FSH in your blood can be a sign that you're transitioning into menopause. Estradiol, on the other hand, tends to decrease as you approach menopause. It's a bit like watching the stock market - if FSH is on the rise and estradiol is dipping, it could be an indication that menopause is underway.

As for the process, it's pretty straightforward. A healthcare provider will draw a small amount of blood from your arm, which is then sent to a lab for analysis. The purpose here is clear - it's about gaining insights into what's happening hormone-wise. Are they throwing a farewell party for your reproductive years, or are they sticking around a bit longer?

Now, you might be wondering, "Do I need a blood test to know if I'm in menopause?" Not necessarily. Many women recognize the signs of menopause and never need a blood test for confirmation. But if your symptoms are ambiguous, or if you're experiencing changes at an unusually early age, hormone blood tests can be instrumental in clarifying the situation.

When are Hormone Blood Tests Recommended?

Hormone blood tests aren't handed out like party favors. They are usually recommended in specific situations. If you're undergoing certain medical treatments like chemotherapy or if you have had your ovaries surgically removed, your doctor might recommend a blood test since these situations can cause menopause-like symptoms.

Moreover, if you're under 45 and have symptoms like irregular or missed periods, hot flashes, night sweats, or any of the other delights of menopause, a hormone blood test could be recommended to determine if you're experiencing early menopause.

Your doctor might also suggest a hormone blood test if you've been using hormonal birth control, which can mask menopause symptoms. If you're on these contraceptives and stop menstruating, it's not always clear whether you're not having periods because of birth control or because you're transitioning into menopause. It's like a hormonal whodunit!

On a final note, remember that blood tests are just one piece of the menopause puzzle. Your doctor may order a variety of tests, and you may simply be in the "normal" range for your age. Normal ranges vary widely, and being in the normal range does not mean you do not have symptoms that need treatment. Your symptoms, health history, and, most importantly, how you feel also play a significant role in piecing together this biological mystery. The more information you have, the more tailored your care plan can be, allowing you to navigate menopause with a clear roadmap. So, whether it's a bit early to say goodbye to your menstrual cycle or you're right on time, remember that you're in the driver's seat, with your healthcare provider as your trusty co-pilot.

EARLY ONSET AND BLOOD TESTS

Ever heard the saying, "The early bird gets the worm?" Well, when it comes to menopause, being the early bird can feel more like being handed a can of worms instead. For those experiencing early onset menopause, there can be a whirlwind of questions, worries, and misinformation. But fear not! Our trusty ally, the blood test, can play a crucial role in understanding and managing this premature plot twist in your hormonal narrative.

Importance of Blood Tests for Women Under 45

Before we dig in, let's establish what early-onset menopause actually is. If your body starts blasting the menopause mixtape before you hit 45, you're officially in the early onset club. It's not the most desirable club to join early, but don't worry – there's no mandatory uniform or secret handshake to learn.

Now, if you're under 45 and you've started experiencing symptoms that hint at menopause (like your periods moonwalking off the regular schedule or hot flashes that would make a dragon feel at home), a blood test can help clear up the confusion. It's like getting a backstage pass to your hormonal concert. Are the headliners – estrogen and progesterone – starting to pack up their instruments? Is FSH warming up for its solo?

Early detection through blood tests can provide a roadmap for managing the symptoms and health risks associated with early menopause. Knowing what's happening in your body can empower you to take steps to protect your heart and bones, both of which can be affected by early menopause. Plus, it gives you a head start on managing the array of symptoms that come with this hormonal transition.

Remember, the complexities of the human body and the myriad ways it can be affected means that menopause isn't the only star of the 'irregular period and hot flash' show. There are other conditions that share the limelight with similar symptoms - think thyroid disorders or certain ovarian conditions. This is why your doctor, who is your partner in this dance, may pull out their detective hat and order a variety of additional tests.

These tests are not about doubting the initial suspicion of early menopause but rather ruling out other potential causes, ensuring that the diagnosis is as accurate as a dart thrown by a world champion. It's about turning over every stone, looking in every nook and cranny, and ensuring nothing else is causing your symptoms.

From a comprehensive thyroid panel to a pelvic ultrasound, these tests can help draw a complete picture of what's happening inside your body. The goal here isn't just to put a name to your condition but to understand its nature, its triggers, and its effects. Only then can you and your doctor craft a strategy that's as unique as your fingerprint, guiding you through early menopause with minimal fuss and maximal grace.

In essence, consider these tests as part of your wellness squad - they're there to ensure you get the most accurate diagnosis, which, in turn, leads to the most effective game plan. It's like playing chess with every piece on the board instead of just the pawns.

Detecting and Managing Early Changes

So, how do we detect these early changes? And, more importantly, how do we manage them? Once again, hormone blood tests come to the rescue. By measuring levels of FSH and estradiol in your blood, your healthcare provider can help determine if you're in the early stages of menopause.

But detecting early changes is just the first part of the story. The sequel is all about managing these changes. If you've got the confirmation that you're experiencing early menopause, it's not about sounding the panic alarms - it's about planning and adapting.

Think of it like being given the heads-up that a heatwave is coming. You wouldn't just stand there, waiting to melt. You'd prepare: stock up on sunblock, invest in some good fans, and maybe even splurge on that air conditioner you've been eyeing. Similarly, getting a heads up on early menopause allows you to take preventative measures to protect your health, like boosting your calcium and vitamin D intake for bone health or making lifestyle changes to support heart health.

And remember, while going through menopause earlier than expected might feel isolating, you're not alone. Lean on your healthcare provider for advice and support, and don't hesitate to reach out to support groups. It's your concert, and you're the main act, but you've got a whole crew ready to help you rock this performance.

CONTRACEPTION CONSIDERATIONS

Contraception helps us navigate the labyrinth of family planning. It's like the satnav of the reproductive world, right? But what happens when we hit that menopausal roadblock? Is it an immediate stop, or do we gently slow down? And how does it impact our hormone test drive? Let's put on our detective hats and figure it out.

Impact of Hormonal Contraception on Blood Tests

So, you're taking hormonal contraception, be it in the form of pills, patches, or injections, and you're curious about how it might influence your hormone blood tests. Well, if hormones were secret agents, contraceptives would be their disguises, altering their identity and making it tricky for us to recognize them. Simply put, hormonal contraception can affect the levels of estrogen and progesterone in your body, which can muddy the waters when it comes to blood tests.

For instance, your doctor might be looking for a decrease in estrogen levels, one of the telltale signs of menopause. However, most hormonal contraceptives contain synthetic forms of estrogen and progesterone, effectively keeping these levels steady. It's like trying to find Wally in a crowd when he's decided to ditch the red and white for a brilliant disguise!

This is not to say that you're in an unsolvable predicament. Doctors can still identify menopause in women using hormonal contraception, but it might require additional tests or strategies.

Guidelines on When to Stop Contraception

One of the most common questions that arise when navigating the choppy waters of menopause is when to stop using contraception. Here's the deal: Menopause is like that one elusive guest at a party – everyone knows they'll show up eventually, but no one quite knows when. And with menopause, the stakes are a bit higher than with a tardy party-goer.

So, when do you bid adieu to your contraceptives? You might be expecting a specific age, but that's like predicting when the next plot twist in your favorite series will occur. It varies. Current guidelines suggest women continue using contraception for a year after their last period if they're over 50 and for two years if they're under 50.

Why the extended timeline, you ask? Well, the eggs in your ovaries might be getting ready to clock off, but occasionally, they pull an overtime shift. These instances of late ovulation could lead to an unexpected pregnancy if contraception is stopped too soon.

Remember, these guidelines are general advice. Your own decision about when to stop contraception should always be made in consultation with your healthcare provider.

KEY TAKEAWAYS

1. Menopause is a natural life event, not an illness. While modern medicine can assist with symptom management, it's not a one-size-fits-all solution.
2. Regular check-ups with your OB-GYN, keeping a symptom diary, and personalized care approach are crucial during menopause.
3. Hormone blood tests help in determining your menopause stage and are particularly vital for women under 45 to detect early onset.
4. Contraception considerations are important during menopause, as hormonal contraception can affect blood test results, and guidelines suggest continuing contraception for a period after the last menstrual cycle.
5. Above all, keep an open dialogue with your healthcare provider, and remember - you're not alone in this journey.

FINAL THOUGHTS

As we dock our menopause ship at the end of this chapter, I want to remind you that you're not just a passenger in this journey—you're the captain. You're steering your course, adjusting your sails, and weathering the occasional storm. And just as every ship needs a good crew, remember that you have a team of experts, from your OB-GYN to other healthcare providers, ready to help.

Navigating through the rough seas of menopause can be daunting, but remember – this is not a storm to be weathered alone. Seek advice, ask questions, and always keep an open line with your healthcare provider. Your menopause experience is as unique as you are and requires personalized care and attention.

And while menopause is a significant life event, it is just that, a part of life, not an illness or something to be 'cured'. The goal of any treatment, whether modern medicine or natural remedies, is not to reverse the process, but to make the journey more comfortable, ensuring you feel empowered and confident every step of the way.

In our next chapter, we'll sail into the fascinating world of natural medicine. So hold tight, and let's explore another way to navigate the menopausal seas.

HARNESSING THE POWER OF NATURE: MANAGING MENOPAUSE SYMPTOMS NATURALLY

Let's ditch the lab coat for a while and embrace the natural, the wholesome, and the nutritious in our journey through menopause. Now, before you start picturing yourself chanting in a forest or foraging for wild herbs, let me assure you: I'll be keeping our feet on the ground, though a little tree hugging never hurt anybody!

As we navigate the turbulent seas of "the change," it's important to remember we have a veritable treasure trove of natural remedies and strategies at our disposal. Menopause might feel like a hot flash-infused cocktail of night sweats, mood swings, and unsolicited weight gain, but it's not all gloom and doom. In this chapter, I'll explore the power of lifestyle choices, dive into the soup of supplements, decode the mystery of vitamins, and reveal the secrets of alternative medicine.

I'll also look at proven coping strategies, so you can not only survive the menopausal roller coaster but thrive on it. Think of it as your handy survival guide, equipping you to ward off the menopause monsters under your bed...or in your bed if night sweats are your main nemesis.

IMPORTANCE OF SUPPLEMENTS DURING MENOPAUSE

Let's talk supplements. Think of them as your secret weapons during the menopause years, but remember they are not substitutes for a balanced diet. They are just there to fill in the nutritional gaps, not replace entire meals. Well, unless your idea of a balanced diet is a slice of pizza in each hand – in which case, we may need to chat.

But why do supplements matter?

Well, as estrogen takes a nosedive during menopause, your body starts acting like a petulant teenager who didn't get invited to the popular kids' party. Hot flashes, night sweats, mood swings – you know, the usual fun stuff. This hormonal transition can affect your body's ability to absorb certain nutrients efficiently, hence the need for some supplementation. But remember, it's not about popping pills willy-nilly. It's about creating balance.

Here are some necessary nutrients with which you may need to supplement your diet:

Magnesium

Think of magnesium as that multi-talented friend we all secretly envy. It's involved in over 300 enzymatic reactions in the body, from nerve function and muscle contraction to blood sugar control and blood pressure regulation. Talk about an overachiever.

During menopause, our superstar friend magnesium can help combat some symptoms. Research indicates that it may improve mood, reduce water retention and bloat, and even help with sleep disturbances. Who needs sheep-counting when you've got magnesium, right?

But, like any good thing, there's always a potential downside. Overdoing magnesium supplementation can lead to cramps, nausea, and even irregular heart rhythms in extreme cases. So, follow the Goldilocks principle – not too much, not too little, but just right.

Vitamin A

Next on our list is Vitamin A, another important guest at our menopause party. This fat-soluble vitamin is crucial for maintaining good vision (no, it won't help you find your reading glasses, but it'll definitely help you see better when you do). It also plays a critical role in supporting the immune system and maintaining healthy skin.

There's some evidence suggesting that vitamin A can help maintain healthy mucous membranes, which can, in turn, alleviate some pesky menopausal symptoms like vaginal dryness. However, before you start chugging vitamin A supplements like there's no tomorrow, let me drop a reality check. Over-supplementing on vitamin A can be harmful and lead to toxicity, which can cause a whole array of problems like dizziness, nausea, and even hair loss. So, as with any supplement, it's about finding the right balance.

Vitamins B6 and B12

Vitamins B6 and B12 are like the dynamic duo of the B-vitamin family. They're Batman and Robin, Thelma and Louise, peanut butter and jelly. Together, they've got your back when it comes to promoting brain health and supporting nerve function. But they're also essential for helping your body convert food into energy, making them a crucial part of the diet, especially during menopause.

B6, a.k.a. Pyridoxine, might have a shy name, but it doesn't shy away from heavy lifting. Studies have found it can help combat depressive symptoms linked with menopause and, in some cases, even alleviate hot flashes.

B12, on the other hand, is the life of the party in nerve cells and red blood cell production. This water-soluble vitamin has a reputation for reducing fatigue, improving memory, and even cheering up your mood.

However, always remember that even superheroes have their kryptonite. Overdoing B6 can lead to nerve damage, while too much B12 can cause side effects like dizziness, headache, anxiety, and nausea.

Vitamin K

Next up, the underrated superhero, Vitamin K. Not just for stopping nosebleeds, Vitamin K is also critical for bone health. Research suggests that it may play a role in maintaining bone density in postmenopausal women, helping prevent osteoporosis. Plus, it supports healthy blood clotting. So, essentially, Vitamin K is the friend who stops you from bleeding out but also makes sure you don't bruise like a peach every time you bump into something.

But don't rush to start popping Vitamin K pills just yet. Too much of it can interfere with blood-thinning medications and can also lead to blood clotting issues. So, if you're on any medication, check with your doctor first.

Vitamin C

Finally, we come to the superstar, Vitamin C. This is the A-lister of the vitamin world, the vitamin everyone's heard of, the vitamin everyone wants at their party. And for a good reason. It's a powerful antioxidant, crucial for skin health, iron absorption, and boosting the immune system. Some studies have also found it may help manage stress and reduce hot flashes in menopausal women.

But before you go reaching for that Vitamin C supplement, remember even superstars have their limits. Too much can lead to diarrhea, nausea, and stomach cramps. As with all things, balance is key.

Calcium

Let's roll out the red carpet for calcium, the rockstar mineral that's been headlining your health ever since you were busy losing baby teeth. Your mom wasn't just throwing old wives' tales around when she told you to finish your milk for strong bones and teeth.

As you gracefully age into your menopause years (or, as we like to call it, your 'fine wine' phase), your body's production of estrogen, a hormone that assists in maintaining bone mass, takes a nosedive. Here's where calcium steps up, plugging the gap and maintaining the integrity of your skeletal system. So, you can continue rocking those heels or go on those long-awaited mountain hikes without worrying about brittle bones.

But like any headliner with an oversized ego, too much calcium isn't all autographs and applause. An overload can lead to constipation or, worse, kidney stones. Nobody wants a backstage pass to that show.

Vitamin D

To get the best performance from calcium, you need its faithful sidekick – Vitamin D, the 'sunshine' vitamin. Vitamin D helps your body absorb calcium, making it indispensable for bone health. Plus, it also plays a role in maintaining your immune function and reducing inflammation.

Unfortunately, as with real sunshine, there can be too much of a good thing. While Vitamin D is busy signing autographs, remember not to overdo it. Excess intake can lead to nausea, vomiting, muscle weakness, and kidney problems.

Omega-3s

Last but definitely not least, let's welcome Omega-3s onto the stage. Omega-3 fatty acids are like the indie musicians of the nutrient world -- they might not be as well-known as some of the mainstream acts, but they certainly know how to put on a show.

These unsaturated fats have been proven to help reduce heart disease risk. They also come in handy in the fight against menopausal symptoms such as hot flashes and night sweats. And for the grand finale, they contribute to the health of your brain and eyes. Talk about a multitasker!

But remember, no encore is needed for Omega-3s. Too much of this supplement can cause nausea, loose stools, and nose-bleeds. Also, they may interact with blood-thinning medications, leading to an increased risk of bleeding.

Probiotics

So you've heard of antibiotics, but what about probiotics? Think of them as the yin to antibiotics' yang. While antibiotics are the bad-boy rockstars smashing their guitars on stage (i.e., killing bacteria), probiotics are the smooth jazz players, calmly restoring order to the place. They're the live "good" bacteria and yeasts that keep your gut healthy, and as it turns out, a happy gut means a happier you during menopause.

Probiotics have been shown to help with digestion, boost immunity, and even improve mental health. And while menopause is turning your hormone world into a mosh pit, probiotics can potentially help manage weight gain and reduce cholesterol levels. That's music to our ears!

But, just like too much jazz can have you falling asleep mid-song, too many probiotics can have some downsides, including bloating and upset stomach. So, moderate your intake – this isn't a probiotic all-nighter!

Turmeric

And now, for our grand finale, let's hear it for the golden child of the spice world – Turmeric! Known for its potent anti-inflammatory properties, this humble spice has been stealing the spotlight in recent years. And rightly so! Its active ingredient, curcumin, is like the Beyoncé of the nutrient world: highly talented and full of surprises. From reducing joint pain to improving brain function and even alleviating menopausal symptoms like hot flashes and mood swings – this superstar has you covered.

Remember, though, turmeric is a strong spice, and like any diva, too much can lead to an upset stomach and even exacerbate gallbladder problems. So, while it can be tempting to drown your curries in this golden goodness, you might want to resist the urge.

Precautions and Possible Interactions with Other Medications

Supplementing your diet with vitamins and minerals during menopause necessitates careful consideration. It is crucial to understand that all these nutrients need to work harmoniously with each other and, most importantly, with any other medication you may be currently using.

For instance, Vitamin K, while beneficial, can influence the effectiveness of blood thinners. Omega-3s, although generally excellent for heart health, may not be compatible with blood pressure medications. Similarly, turmeric, despite its numerous health benefits, can have adverse interactions with medications such as aspirin and warfarin.

The key takeaway is to exercise caution. Always consult your healthcare provider before introducing new supplements into your routine, especially if you're currently taking other medications. Your menopause journey is a personal one, and it's essential to ensure that all elements work together for optimal health and well-being.

NATURAL REMEDIES

Natural remedies for menopause aren't just age-old wisdom passed down from your grandma's grandma; they're strategies steeped in scientific research.

"Why consider natural remedies?" you ask. Well, while traditional pharmaceuticals target symptoms with precision, they can sometimes bring along unwelcome side effects. Natural remedies, on the other hand, aim to work in sync with your body, gently nudging it back toward balance. They might take a bit longer to show effects, but their aim is holistic well-being.

Remember though, natural doesn't always mean 'side-effect-free'. Depending on your health, some natural remedies may work better for you than others. It's all about finding what fits your unique menopausal puzzle!

Role of Phytoestrogens

Now, if you've hung around health circles or stumbled upon a forum discussing menopause, you've probably come across the term "phytoestrogens". And you might think, "Oh great, another weird-named compound. What's it going to do, summon a phyto-goddess to end my menopausal misery?" Well, you might not be too far off.

Phytoestrogens, despite their mouthful name, are exciting compounds found in various foods, especially soy and flaxseeds. They are the chameleons of the natural compounds world - they can mimic the hormone estrogen in your body. It's like having a stand-in for your favorite band's lead singer - not the real deal, but hey, the show must go on!

During menopause, your body's estrogen production dwindles, leaving you with a series of uncomfortable symptoms. This is where phytoestrogens step in – they put on their estrogen costumes and help fill the void, easing symptoms such as hot flashes, mood swings, and night sweats.

But let's not get carried away. While they may seem like your knight in shining armor, phytoestrogens come with their own baggage. The research is split – while some studies found them to reduce hot flashes, others suggest they have no significant impact. There are even concerns about their safety in women with a high risk of estrogen-sensitive cancers, like breast cancer.

If you're thinking of adding phytoestrogens to your menopausal regimen, it's crucial to have a chat with your healthcare provider.

Unveiling the Super Four: Black Cohosh, Red Clover, Dong Quai, and Ginseng

Let's kick off this section by introducing our power quartet. Think of them as the Beatles of natural menopause remedies: Black Cohosh, Red Clover, Dong Quai, and Ginseng. Just as each band member brought something unique to their music, each of these plants provides different potential benefits for menopausal symptoms.

Black Cohosh - The Enigmatic Diva

Black Cohosh has been a regular on the menopausal relief charts for years and for good reason. Multiple studies suggest it might help ease hot flashes and night sweats. One meta-analysis published in The Obstetrician & Gynaecologist reviewed 16 trials and concluded that Black Cohosh could be an effective alternative for reducing hot flashes compared to a placebo. Now that's music to our ears!

However, our diva has a downside. Some studies report possible liver damage with extended use of Black Cohosh, but these cases are very rare. And, as with any supplement or remedy, it's essential to follow the recommended dosage.

Red Clover - The Cool Bassist

Red Clover is all about heart health and bone strength. Research published in the journal Menopause found that women who took Red Clover supplements had a slower progression of arterial stiffness, a risk factor for heart disease. And as a bonus track, Red Clover might also help improve bone mineral density, reducing the risk of osteoporosis.

However, Red Clover can occasionally hit a sour note. It contains natural compounds that mimic estrogen, so if you have a condition that could be worsened by estrogen—like some breast cancers—you'll want to give Red Clover a miss.

Dong Quai - The Soulful Vocalist

Dong Quai, often referred to as the "female ginseng," has been used in traditional Chinese medicine for thousands of years to help with various health issues, including menopausal symptoms. Its benefits are thought to include easing hot flashes and mood swings.

But here's a cautionary note. Dong Quai can increase your skin's sensitivity to the sun, possibly leading to skin inflammation. It also may interfere with blood clotting, so it's not recommended for those with bleeding disorders or taking blood thinners.

Ginseng - The Versatile Drummer

Ginseng rounds out our band. Its versatility is its strength. From helping manage menopausal symptoms like hot flashes, night sweats, and mood swings to boosting energy levels and cognitive function, Ginseng appears to have it all.

However, ginseng can be a potent stimulant and may cause insomnia in some individuals. Also, those with high blood pressure should approach Ginseng with caution.

Like any good band, each of these plant-based remedies brings its unique flair to the stage. However, it's crucial to note that while they've shown potential in managing menopausal symptoms, more comprehensive, rigorous research is needed. And remember, always consult with your healthcare provider before starting any new supplement regimen.

HOLISTIC WELLNESS APPROACHES

In the journey through menopause, sometimes the most potent remedies are the simple, everyday choices we make. This section explores these natural lifestyle adjustments that can effectively mitigate menopausal symptoms. The goal here is not only to manage your menopausal symptoms but also to enhance your overall health and well-being during this significant life phase. Let's get started.

Delving Deeper into the World of Balanced Diet for Menopausal Women

In Chapter 4, we nibbled around the edges of the diet topic like we were at a fancy cocktail party with an hors d'oeuvres tray. But now, it's time to sit down for the full-course meal. Let's get into the nitty-gritty of why a balanced diet is so essential during menopause, breaking it down course by course.

Avoiding Trigger Foods – Navigating the Dietary Minefield

During menopause, your body may suddenly start reacting differently to foods and beverages you've enjoyed without issue for years. These culinary culprits can bring on those inconvenient hot flashes and capricious mood swings. In the crosshairs often stand alcohol, caffeine, and spicy foods. In fact, a study published in the Menopause Journal found a correlation between these substances and an increase in hot flashes and night sweats.

However, everyone's menopausal journey is unique. What triggers unpleasant symptoms in one woman may have no effect on another. This makes it vital for you to monitor your body's reactions to different foods and beverages. Keeping a food diary might be a handy way to track these responses, giving you a personalized guide to the foods and drinks that spark your symptoms.

In practice, avoiding trigger foods can mean tweaking some of your eating habits. Are you a coffee lover who can't do without your morning cup? Try decaf or caffeinated tea instead. Do you love spicing things up in your meals? Experiment with herbs and other flavors that don't turn up the heat. A little patience and creativity can go a long way in helping you navigate this dietary minefield.

Cutting Down Refined Sugar and Processed Foods – Your Health's Secret Weapon

Refined sugars and processed foods are masterful at flying under the radar. They're often hidden in unsuspecting places like sauces, low-fat foods, and beverages, carrying high caloric content and offering low nutritional value in return. This stealthy combination can contribute to weight gain and an increased risk of heart disease. Moreover, the high glycemic index of these foods can lead to rapid spikes and falls in blood sugar levels, resulting in energy crashes and increased hunger.

According to a study in the American Journal of Clinical Nutrition, diets high in processed foods and sugars are associated with increased risks of chronic diseases. This doesn't mean you must completely ban these foods from your diet, but moderation is key. Begin by checking labels for hidden sugars, opt for whole foods whenever possible, and try substituting natural sugars like fruits for your sweet cravings.

Additionally, cutting down on these foods helps maintain a healthy gut microbiome, an often overlooked aspect of overall health. Imbalances in gut bacteria can lead to inflammation and other health issues. So, it's not an exaggeration to say that reducing refined sugars and processed foods is a secret weapon in managing your menopausal symptoms and promoting overall health.

Fruits and Vegetables – Harnessing the Power of Plant-Based Foods

If there ever was a culinary superhero team to tackle menopause, fruits, and vegetables would be it. They're bursting with vitamins, minerals, and fiber, which are all vital for general health and well-being. More importantly, several fruits and veggies are high in antioxidants, which can help combat the oxidative stress that exacerbates menopausal symptoms.

A study published in the *American Journal of Epidemiology* found that women who consumed a diet rich in vegetables, fruit, and fiber had a 19% lower risk of experiencing hot flashes. Plus, a separate study in the journal *Menopause* confirmed that a higher intake of fruits and vegetables is associated with a lower prevalence of menopausal symptoms.

But the benefits of these plant powerhouses don't stop there. Many fruits and veggies are also low in calories and high in fiber, which can help manage weight—a common issue during menopause. In essence, making fruits and vegetables a primary part of your meals can help you load up on nutrients without piling on the pounds.

Calcium and Vitamin D – The Guardians of Bone Health

During menopause, your body's production of estrogen—a hormone crucial for bone health—takes a nosedive. This leads to an increased rate of bone loss, raising the risk of osteoporosis. Enter calcium and vitamin D, the guardian angels of your skeletal system during menopause.

Calcium is the primary nutrient responsible for strong, healthy bones. But it's vitamin D that allows your body to effectively absorb this essential mineral. In short, they're a dynamic duo working together for your benefit. According to the National Osteoporosis Foundation, adult women should aim for 1,200mg of calcium and 800-1,000 IU of vitamin D daily.

Foods rich in these nutrients include dairy products, fortified cereals, and oily fish. And let's not forget sunlight—it's a prime source of vitamin D! A study published in *The Journal of the American College of Nutrition* revealed that a combination of calcium and vitamin D has the potential to slow the rate of bone loss in menopausal women, thus reducing the risk of fractures.

Maintaining a Moderate Weight – The Balancing Act

Menopause often brings with it a shift in body composition and distribution of fat. The fluctuation of hormones can slow down your metabolism, leading to weight gain. This doesn't just affect your wardrobe choices; it also increases the risk of health issues like heart disease and diabetes.

Maintaining a moderate weight through a balanced diet and regular exercise can be one of the best things you do for your health during menopause. According to research published in Menopause, women who had a healthy body weight were less likely to experience severe menopausal symptoms.

This doesn't mean embarking on a drastic diet or exercise regimen. Small, sustainable changes often yield the best results. This can be as simple as choosing whole grains over refined ones, drinking plenty of water, and finding physical activities that you genuinely enjoy. Remember, the goal here isn't to attain a specific number on the scale but to nurture a healthier, happier you through this transition.

Physical Activity

Working out is like doing your body a series of mini-favors. It's not just about losing weight or building muscle - it's about investing in your overall health. Regular exercise can help reduce the risk of heart disease, diabetes, and several types of cancer. But the benefits are not just physical. Breaking a sweat can also help improve your mood and boost your self-esteem. After all, endorphins make you happy, and happy people just don't shoot their husbands, right?

When it comes to menopause, a study published in *Menopause Review* found that regular exercise helped manage menopausal symptoms like hot flashes and night sweats, along with improving bone health and reducing the risk of breast cancer.

So, now you know why you should exercise, but what kind of exercise should you do? Like a buffet, there's a wide range of exercises to choose from, each with its benefits.

Cardio exercises such as jogging, swimming, or cycling can help keep your heart healthy and manage weight. Strength training is excellent for bone health, and it can help manage the changes in body composition that occur during menopause. And let's not forget flexibility exercises like yoga and Pilates, which can help keep you agile and manage stress.

The important thing is to find something that you love doing. After all, exercise shouldn't feel like punishment. It should be a celebration of what your body can do.

Hydration

Drinking enough water is crucial for your overall health. It's like oil for your body's engine—it helps everything run smoothly. Water aids in digestion, absorption of nutrients, circulation, and even temperature control.

But what's the role of water in menopause? Hot flashes, night sweats, and other menopausal symptoms can lead to increased water loss. Therefore, keeping yourself hydrated is key in managing these symptoms. A study in the journal *Menopause* found that hydration can help maintain the skin's elasticity, which often decreases during menopause.

Consuming Phytoestrogen-Rich Foods

Now, let's talk about phytoestrogens. No, they're not a new indie rock band. They're plant-derived compounds that function similarly to the estrogen in our bodies.

Phytoestrogens can be particularly beneficial during menopause. With the decrease in estrogen levels during this time, these plant-derived compounds can help fill the void. They can help manage symptoms like hot flashes and night sweats, and according to a review in *The Journal of Steroid Biochemistry and Molecular Biology*, they may even play a role in preventing osteoporosis.

So where can you find these mighty compounds? There are several delicious and nutritious foods you can add to your menu:

- Soy products: tofu, tempeh, soy milk, and edamame
- Flaxseeds
- Sesame seeds
- Berries: strawberries, cranberries, and raspberries
- Whole grains: oats, barley, and brown rice
- Vegetables: garlic, celery, and beans

Before introducing any new foods into your diet, especially if you have allergies or are on medication, it's always a good idea to consult with your healthcare provider. They can guide you on the best dietary choices for your personal needs and lifestyle.

KEY TAKEAWAYS

1. Menopause, while challenging, is a natural life stage, and proper nutritional choices can significantly manage symptoms.

2. A balanced diet, including regular meals rich in protein, fruits, vegetables, and foods high in calcium and vitamin D, can support your health during menopause.

3. Physical activity tailored to your preference and capacity can provide both physical and mental health benefits, including managing menopausal symptoms.

4. Staying well-hydrated and including phytoestrogen-rich foods in your diet can further aid in managing menopausal symptoms.

5. Always consult with your healthcare provider before making significant dietary changes or introducing new supplements or natural remedies.

FINAL THOUGHTS

Navigating menopause might feel like traversing an untamed wilderness, but remember, you hold the compass. It's your journey, and you get to decide how to travel through it. Armed with knowledge and a proactive approach, you can turn this chapter of life into a time of self-discovery and renewal.

Menopause isn't a pause on life but a pivot, an opportunity to focus on your health, your happiness, and your dreams. Start with these actionable tips—nourishing your body with the right foods, moving it with joy, hydrating it, and embracing nature's bounty—to lay a strong foundation for a positive menopause journey.

Remember, this isn't just about surviving menopause—it's about thriving, reclaiming your power, and continuing to write your narrative, with every new day an opportunity to pen an exciting new chapter. So, keep this knowledge close and let it guide you as you navigate the path of menopause with grace, resilience, and optimism.

AFTERWORD

"My mission in life is not merely to survive, but to thrive; and to do so with some passion, some compassion, some humor, and some style."
Maya Angelou

In our exploration through this book, we've danced with the intricacies of menopause, stepping in time with the hormonal symphony and learning to take the lead when needed. From demystifying the whirlwind of symptoms to understanding the myriad of solutions nature and science offer us, we've unpacked menopause, one hot flash and night sweat at a time.

Menopause is often seen as a tricky mid-life plot twist, but really, it's your own personal superhero movie. You've navigated through the ups and downs, faced villains named Anxiety and Mood Swings, and learned how to fuel your superpowers with the right foods, supplements, and a dash of self-love. The cape's been there all along; now you know how to wear it.

We've also learned that there's a kind of magic in menopause, a kind you might not have expected. This phase of life isn't about stepping back; it's about stepping into your own. It's about reclaiming power, harnessing strength, and embracing change. Like a fine wine, life only gets better with time, and ladies, we're just getting started.

Our journey, filled with a few laughs, some hard truths, and plenty of empowering moments, has given us something precious: Knowledge. Knowledge that sparks courage instills resilience and turns the menopause narrative on its head. We've moved from surviving to thriving, and that's a shift worth celebrating.

Remember, dear reader, this is your journey. It's about finding what works for you. Advocate for yourself, experiment, and find your balance. Reach out for that piece of dark chocolate if it makes your day, take that evening walk if it clears your head, sing at the top of your lungs if it sets your spirit free. After all, menopause isn't a malady to be feared; it's a melody to be played, and you're the maestro.

Now, take this wisdom, this beautiful blend of science, nature, and soulful insights, and put it to work. Paint the canvas of your life with vibrant colors of health and happiness. Try everything, laugh often, nurture yourself, and always keep dancing to the rhythm of life.

As you embark on this new chapter of your life, remember to always embrace yourself with kindness. You've weathered the hormonal roller-coaster, now it's time to enjoy the calm and wisdom that follows the storm. Menopause is not a pause; it's an exclamation point, a declaration of strength, resilience, and undying spirit.

If this book has resonated with you, consider recommending this read to a comrade in "menopause arms" by leaving a review on Amazon. Share your thoughts, your breakthroughs, and your laughter, and let other warriors know they're not alone.

Now, armed with the gift of knowledge, go out there and seize the day. It's your time to shine, to lead, to inspire. Remember, you're not just surviving menopause; you're thriving through it, and there's nothing more powerful than that.

BIBLIOGRAPHY

A closer look at hormone replacement therapy for menopause. (2023, May 17). [Video]. NBC News. https://www.nbcnews.com/health/womens-health/hot-flashes-treatment-fda-clears-nonhormonal-drug-night-sweats-rcna84025

Bioidentical hormones: Are they safer? (2022, December 7). Mayo Clinic. https://www.mayoclinic.org/diseases-conditions/menopause/expert-answers/bioidentical-hormones/faq-20058460

Black Cohosh. (n.d.). NCCIH. https://www.nccih.nih.gov/health/black-cohosh

Bottaro, A. (2022). *Can hair loss be a symptom of menopause?* Verywell Health. https://www.verywellhealth.com/menopause-hair-loss-5218350

Bowers, P. (2023). *Mind over menopause: Lose Weight, Love Your Body, and Embrace Life After 50 with a Powerful New Mindset.* Experiment.

Can menopause cause depression? (2021, August 8). Johns Hopkins Medicine. https://www.hopkinsmedicine.org/health/wellness-and-prevention/can-menopause-cause-depression

Carmody, J., Crawford, S. L., Salmoirago-Blotcher, E., Leung, K., Churchill, L. C., & Olendzki, N. (2011). *Mindfulness training for coping with hot flashes.* Menopause, 18(6), 611–620. https://doi.org/10.1097/gme.0b013e318204a05c

Carpenter, J. S., Gass, M., Maki, P. M., Newton, K. M., Pinkerton, J. V., Taylor, M., Utian, W. H., Schnatz, P. F., Kaunitz, A. M., Shapiro, M., Shifren, J. L., Hodis, H. N., Kingsberg, S. A., Liu, J. H., Richard-Davis, G., Santoro, N., Sievert, L. L., Schiff, I., & Pike, C. (2015). *Nonhormonal management of menopause-associated vasomotor symptoms.* Menopause, 22(11), 1155–1174. https://doi.org/10.1097/gme.0000000000000546

Changes in Hormone Levels, Sexual Side Effects of Menopause | The North American Menopause Society, NAMS. (n.d.). https://www.menopause. org/for-women/sexual-health-menopause-online/changes-at-midlife/ changes-in-hormone-levels

Cramer, H., Peng, W., & Lauche, R. (2018). *Yoga for menopausal symptoms —A systematic review and meta-analysis.* Maturitas, 109, 13–25. https://doi.org/10.1016/j.maturitas.2017.12.005

Dalziel, E. (2023, February 9). *All women who reach their 50s inevitably pass through menopause. Experts share the latest science and best ways to cope.* National Geographic. https://www.nationalgeographic.co.uk/science- and-technology/2023/02/what-happens-during-menopause-science-is- finally-piecing-it-together

Delamater, L., & Santoro, N. (2018). *Management of the perimenopause.* Clinical Obstetrics and Gynecology, 61(3), 419–432. https://doi.org/ 10.1097/grf.0000000000000389

Department of Health & Human Services. (n.d.-a). *Menopause and complementary therapies.* Better Health Channel. https://www.better health.vic.gov.au/health/conditionsandtreatments/menopause-and- complementary-therapies

Department of Health & Human Services. (n.d.-b). *Menopause and weight.* Better Health Channel. https://www.betterhealth.vic.gov.au/health/ conditionsandtreatments/menopause-and-weight-gain

Dodin, S., Blanchet, C., Marc, I., Ernst, E., Wu, T., Vaillancourt, C., Paquette, J., & Maunsell, E. (2013). *Acupuncture for menopausal hot flushes.* The Cochrane Library. https://doi.org/10.1002/14651858. cd007410.pub2

Ee, C., Xue, C. C., Chondros, P., Myers, S. P., French, S., Teede, H., & Pirotta, M. (2016). *Acupuncture for menopausal hot flashes.* Annals of Internal Medicine, 164(3), 146. https://doi.org/10.7326/m15-1380

Elkins, G., Fisher, W., Johnson, A., Carpenter, J. S., & Keith, T. Z. (2013). *Clinical hypnosis in the treatment of postmenopausal hot flashes.* Menopause, 20(3), 291–298. https://doi.org/10.1097/gme.

0b013e31826ce3ed

Files, J. A., Ko, M. G., & Pruthi, S. (2011). *Bioidentical hormone therapy*. Mayo Clinic Proceedings, 86(7), 673–680. https://doi.org/10.4065/mcp.2010.0714

George, R. (2017, November 29). *What science doesn't know about the menopause: what it's for and how to treat it*. The Guardian. https://www.theguardian.com/society/2015/dec/15/what-science-doesnt-know-about-the-menopause-what-its-for-how-to-treat-it

Gersh, F., & Perella, A. (2021). *Menopause: 50 Things You Need to Know: What to Expect During the Three Stages of Menopause*. Rockridge Press.

Gunter, J. (2021). *The Menopause Manifesto: Own Your Health with Facts and Feminism*. Random House Canada.

Herbal Remedies for Menopause, Menopause Information & Articles | The North American Menopause Society, NAMS. (n.d.). https://www.menopause.org/for-women/menopauseflashes/menopause-symptoms-and-treatments/natural-remedies-for-hot-flashes

How sex changes after Menopause. (2021, November 10). Johns Hopkins Medicine. https://www.hopkinsmedicine.org/health/wellness-and-prevention/how-sex-changes-after-menopause

How to know if you're going through perimenopause. (2023, May 16). Planned Parenthood. https://www.plannedparenthood.org/blog/how-to-know-if-youre-going-through-perimenopause

Johnson, A., Roberts, R. L., & Elkins, G. (2019). *Complementary and alternative medicine for menopause*. Journal of Evidence-based Integrative Medicine, 24, 2515690X1982938. https://doi.org/10.1177/2515690x19829380

Kantrowitz, B., & Wingert, P. (2018). *The Menopause Book: The Complete Guide: Hormones, Hot Flashes, Health, Moods, Sleep, Sex*. Workman Publishing.

Kaput, K. (2023, June 29). *Supplements for Menopause symptoms: Are they safe?* Cleveland Clinic. https://health.clevelandclinic.org/menopause-supplements/

Kelley, K. W., & Carroll, D. G. (2010). *Evaluating the evidence for over-the-counter alternatives for relief of hot flashes in menopausal women.* Journal of the American Pharmacists Association, 50(5), e106–e115. https://doi.org/10.1331/japha.2010.09243

Koyuncu T, Unsal A, Arslantas D. *Evaluation of the Effectiveness of Health Education on Menopause Symptoms and Knowledge and Attitude in Terms of Menopause.* J Epidemiol Glob Health. 2018 Dec;8(1-2):8-12. doi: 10.2991/j.jegh.2018.08.103. PMID: 30859781; PMCID: PMC7325820.

Lipold, L., Batur, P., & Kagan, R. (2016). *Is there a time limit for systemic menopausal hormone therapy?* Cleveland Clinic Journal of Medicine. https://doi.org/10.3949/ccjm.83a.15161

Management of menopausal symptoms. (n.d.). ACOG. https://www.acog.org/clinical/clinical-guidance/practice-bulletin/articles/2014/01/management-of-menopausal-symptoms

McDermott, A. (2023, June 26). *Can vitamins help alleviate my menopause symptoms?* Healthline. https://www.healthline.com/health/menopause/vitamins-for-menopause

Mehta, J., Kling, J. M., & Manson, J. E. (2021). *Risks, benefits, and treatment modalities of Menopausal hormone therapy: Current concepts.* Frontiers in Endocrinology, 12. https://doi.org/10.3389/fendo.2021.564781

Menopausal symptoms and complementary health approaches. (n.d.). NCCIH. https://www.nccih.nih.gov/health/providers/digest/menopausal-symptoms-and-complementary-health-approaches-science

Menopausal symptoms: in depth. (n.d.). NCCIH. https://www.nccih.nih.gov/health/menopausal-symptoms-in-depth

Menopause | Office on Women's Health. (n.d.). https://www.womenshealth.gov/menopause

Menopause - Diagnosis and treatment - Mayo Clinic. (2023a, May 25). https://www.mayoclinic.org/diseases-conditions/menopause/diagnosis-treatment/drc-20353401

Menopause - Diagnosis and treatment - Mayo Clinic. (2023b, May 25). https://www.mayoclinic.org/diseases-conditions/menopause/diagnosis-treatment/drc-20353401

Menopause and your health | Office on Women's Health. (n.d.). https://www.womenshealth.gov/menopause/menopause-and-your-health

Menopause and your mental wellbeing. (n.d.). NHS Inform. https://www.nhsinform.scot/healthy-living/womens-health/later-years-around-50-years-and-over/menopause-and-post-menopause-health/menopause-and-your-mental-wellbeing

Menopause basics | Office on Women's Health. (n.d.). https://www.womenshealth.gov/menopause/menopause-basics

Menopause Hormone Therapy (HT) Benefits & Risks, Menopause Relief | The North American Menopause Society, NAMS. (n.d.). https://www.menopause.org/for-women/menopauseflashes/menopause-symptoms-and-treatments/hormone-therapy-benefits-risks

Minkin, M. J. (2019). *Menopause.* Obstetrics and Gynecology Clinics of North America, 46(3), 501–514. https://doi.org/10.1016/j.ogc.2019.04.008

Mosca, L., Collins, P., Herrington, D. M., Mendelsohn, M. E., Pasternak, R. C., Robertson, R. M., Schenck-Gustafsson, K., Smith, S. C., Taubert, K. A., & Wenger, N. K. (2001). *Hormone replacement therapy and cardiovascular disease.* Circulation, 104(4), 499–503. https://doi.org/10.1161/hc2901.092200

Natural Treatments for Menopause Symptoms. (2006, December 31). WebMD. https://www.webmd.com/menopause/menopause-natural-treatments

Newson, L. (2023). *The Definitive Guide to the Perimenopause and Menopause.* Yellow Kite.

Office of the Commissioner. (2019a). *Menopause.* U.S. Food And Drug Administration. https://www.fda.gov/consumers/womens-health-topics/menopause

Office of the Commissioner. (2019b). *Menopause: Medicines to help you.* U.S. Food And Drug Administration. https://www.fda.gov/consumers/free-publications-women/menopause-medicines-help-you

Office of the Commissioner. (2023). *FDA approves novel drug to treat moderate to severe hot flashes caused by menopause. U.S. Food And Drug Administration.* https://www.fda.gov/news-events/press-announce ments/fda-approves-novel-drug-treat-moderate-severe-hot-flashes-caused-menopause

Perimenopause. (2021, August 8). Johns Hopkins Medicine. https://hopkinsmedicine.org/health/conditions-and-diseases/perimenopause

Perimenopause - Symptoms and causes - Mayo Clinic. (2023, May 25). Mayo Clinic. https://www.mayoclinic.org/diseases-conditions/peri menopause/symptoms-causes/syc-20354666

Pinkerton, J. a. V., Aguirre, F. S., Blake, J., Cosman, F., Hodis, H. N., Hoffstetter, S., Kaunitz, A. M., Kingsberg, S. A., Maki, P. M., Manson, J. a. E., Marchbanks, P. A., McClung, M. R., Nachtigall, L. E., Nelson, L. M., Pace, D. T., Reid, R. L., Sarrel, P., Shifren, J. L., Stuenkel, C. A., & Utian, W. H. (2017). *The 2017 hormone therapy position statement of The North American Menopause Society.* Menopause, 24(7), 728–753. https://doi.org/10.1097/gme.0000000000000921

Practice Bulletin No. 141. (2014). Obstetrics & Gynecology, 123(1), 202–216. https://doi.org/10.1097/01.aog.0000441353.20693.78

Professional, C. C. M. (n.d.-a). *Hair loss in women.* Cleveland Clinic. https://my.clevelandclinic.org/health/diseases/16921-hair-loss-in-women

Professional, C. C. M. (n.d.-b). *Hormone therapy for menopause symptoms.* Cleveland Clinic. https://my.clevelandclinic.org/health/treatments/15245-hormone-therapy-for-menopause-symptoms

Professional, C. C. M. (n.d.-c). *Perimenopause.* Cleveland Clinic. https://my.clevelandclinic.org/health/diseases/21608-perimenopause

Rd, M. J. B. P. (2023, April 21). *11 Natural Remedies for Menopause Relief.* Healthline. https://www.healthline.com/nutrition/11-natural-menopause-tips

Sex and Menopause. (2002, October 6). WebMD. https://www.webmd.com/menopause/sex-menopause

Sex and Menopause: Treatment for Symptoms. (n.d.). National Institute on Aging. https://www.nia.nih.gov/health/sex-and-menopause-treatment-symptoms

Sleep problems and menopause: What can I do? (n.d.). National Institute on Aging. https://www.nia.nih.gov/health/sleep-problems-and-menopause-what-can-i-do

Stuenkel, C. A., Davis, S. R., Gompel, A., Lumsden, M. A., Murad, M. H., Pinkerton, J. a. V., & Santen, R. J. (2015). *Treatment of Symptoms of the Menopause: An Endocrine Society Clinical Practice Guideline.* The Journal of Clinical Endocrinology and Metabolism, 100(11), 3975–4011. https://doi.org/10.1210/jc.2015-2236

Süss, H., & Ehlert, U. (2020). *Psychological resilience during the perimenopause.* Maturitas, 131, 48–56. https://doi.org/10.1016/j.maturitas.2019.10.015

The menopause years. (n.d.). ACOG. https://www.acog.org/womens-health/faqs/the-menopause-years

The reality of menopause weight gain. (2023, July 8). Mayo Clinic. https://www.mayoclinic.org/healthy-lifestyle/womens-health/in-depth/menopause-weight-gain/art-20046058

Watson, S. (2014, April 27). *Migraines and menopause.* WebMD. https://www.webmd.com/migraines-headaches/migraines-menopause

Website, N. (2022, May 24). *Things you can do.* nhs.uk. https://www.nhs.uk/conditions/menopause/things-you-can-do/

What are the treatments for other symptoms of menopause? (2021, November 16). https://www.nichd.nih.gov/. https://www.nichd.nih.gov/health/topics/menopause/conditioninfo/treatments

What is menopause? (n.d.). National Institute on Aging. https://www.nia.nih.gov/health/what-menopause

Wierman, M. E., Arlt, W., Basson, R., Davis, S. R., Miller, K. K., Murad, M. H., Rosner, W., & Santoro, N. (2014). *Androgen Therapy in Women: A Reappraisal: An Endocrine Society Clinical Practice Guideline.* The Journal of Clinical Endocrinology and Metabolism, 99(10), 3489–3510. https://doi.org/10.1210/jc.2014-2260

Winona Editorial Team. (2021). *The effects of menopause & how it impacts your brain.* Winona Wellness. https://bywinona.com/journal/the-effects-of-menopause-and-how-it-impacts-your-brain

ABOUT THE AUTHOR

An ardent explorer of the human condition, Lisa M. Carroll is an author who transforms personal adversity into global advocacy. When Lisa's personal encounter with menopause revealed a stark void in accessible, empathetic resources for women, she rose to the challenge. Trading her Air Force uniform for a writer's quill, this retired Judge Advocate embarked on a mission to empower women through knowledge.

Lisa's decade-long journey through perimenopause imbues her writing with authenticity and deep understanding. She artfully weaves her experiences, not just as an author, but as a mother, partner, friend, and self-proclaimed goofball, creating a tapestry that resonates with women everywhere.

Equally at home in a courtroom, an Air Force base, or applying her perfect lipliner, Lisa is as multifaceted as the women she writes for. Through her candid exploration of menopause, Lisa seeks to embolden women to navigate this crucial life stage with confidence and camaraderie. For Lisa M. Carroll, the mission is clear: to ensure no woman faces menopause feeling isolated, unprepared, or misunderstood.

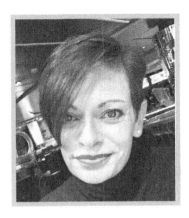

https://www.lisamarycarroll.com

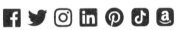

Made in the USA
Monee, IL
03 October 2023